Praise for *Heart Smart for Black Women and Latinas*

"A simple, logical, and achievable three-step plan that can lead you to huge heart-health gains in five weeks. . . . Taking those critical steps will change your life and the lives of those whom you love. Let's start today!"
—Kathy Kastan, L.C.S.W./M.A.Ed., president of WomenHeart and author of
  From the Heart: A Woman's Guide to Living Well with Heart Disease

"This book is an important wake-up call for Black women and Latinas to understand that small steps can make a difference in preventing heart disease. Read this book for yourself and your sisters, but also for your family's good health."
—Nancy Loving, heart-disease survivor and cofounder of WomenHeart

"There's no time like the present to begin your journey toward living a heart-healthy lifestyle. *Heart Smart for Black Women and Latinas* introduces three simple steps that will guide you and your family as you jump-start your journey to living a heart-healthy lifestyle. You will soon see, as I did, that small steps can make a big difference!"
—Vernita Morgan, B.A., doctoral student in Educational Measurement and
  Statistics, the University of Iowa, and a participant in the American Heart
  Association's Choose To Move program

"Rarely does a book come along that not only offers information on what to do but how to do things that can actually save a life. . . . I've known Dr. Jennifer Mieres for years. She and I have often had 'sistah' talks about health issues while sitting side by side under the dryers at our favorite hair salon. Her advice to me when my own sister had a heart attack, thankfully surviving it, was not just meaningful and encouraging but affirming and helped me to understand that heart disease is curable. Now here's a chance for everyone who cares about Black women and Latinas to have that 'sistah' talk with Dr. Mieres. This book is a much-needed guide to heart health for minority women in America today."
—Rehema Ellis, *NBC News* correspondent

"*Heart Smart for Black Women and Latinas* will guide you to a heart-healthy lifestyle by providing simple suggestions for making changes that you can actually incorporate into your busy schedule. It will help you learn how to eat well, get moving, and reduce stress."
—Susan Somerville, R.N., M.A., executive director, North Shore University
  Hospital

"*Heart Smart for Black Women and Latinas* is *the book* that every Black and Latina woman needs to read today. This well-written book will serve as a guide for women who want to prevent heart disease, deal with it if they have it, and how to be proactive about health in general. This is a book with a simple, straightforward message that can help you change your life for the better in a few short weeks.

Start reading this today to take your first step on the road to a healthier and stronger heart!"
—Martha Gulati, M.D., M.S., F.A.C.C., cardiologist, Bluhm Cardiovascular Institute at Northwestern Memorial Hospital's Center for Women's Cardiovascular Health and coauthor of *Heart Power Recipes: Healthy Delicious Whole Food Ideas for the Home Cook*

"*Heart Smart* provides a practical five-week program to get you on your way to living a heart-healthy life—moving more, eating better, stressing less, and enjoying life! It answers all the questions that have gone unanswered for the 'forgotten women.' Many books on heart disease are available to women, but only *Heart Smart* is written for women of color. So get a family member or a friend and begin today to get on the road to heart-healthy living."
—Stacey E. Rosen, M.D., F.A.C.C., chief of Cardiology, Long Island Jewish Medical Center

"*Heart Smart for Black Women and Latinas* will jump-start you on your journey to a healthier lifestyle! I watched my mother prepare food for years, starting with the crackling of lard on a hot pan. I savored refried beans with cheese on flour tortillas, salty fries, crispy *chuletas,* and *huevos con chorizo.* I'm in my late twenties and I'm starting to plan for a family so I decided I needed to become a healthier me. When all your family and friends eat unhealthy foods, it's very easy to ignore or even forget the facts. Living healthy is about more than just diet; it's about reducing calories, burning the extra ones, and adding years to my life because I care for those who love me. *Heart Smart* will help . . . so don't wait another moment. Get your copy of *Heart Smart* today and make yourself a priority."
—Zulema Esparza, schoolteacher and participant in the American Heart Association's Choose To Move program

"This book has the potential to change lives and communities. By breaking down the journey to a healthy heart into small steps, Dr. Mieres and Ms. Parnell make it possible for any woman to live longer and stronger. It should be bedside reading for any woman of color."
—Andrea King Collier, author of *The Black Woman's Guide to Black Men's Health*

A 5-Week Program for Living a Heart-Healthy Lifestyle

Heart
Smart
for Black Women
and Latinas

JENNIFER H. MIERES, M.D., F.A.H.A., *and*
TERRI ANN PARNELL, R.N., M.A.,
with CAROL TURKINGTON

 St. Martin's Griffin *New York*

We dedicate this book to our mothers, sisters, and daughters: Jean Mieres, Terry Quinn, Jacqui Leviton, Jacqueline Mieres-Johnston, Arlene Mieres-Franczak, Aubrey Gershenson, and Zoë Mieres Fleishaker.

www.stmartins.com

Design by Ruth Lee-Mui

ISBN-13: 978-0-312-37267-5
ISBN-10: 0-312-37267-1

First Edition: February 2008

10 9 8 7 6 5 4 3 2 1

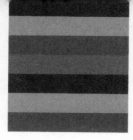

Note to Reader

This book is for informational purposes only. It is not intended to take the place of medical advice from a trained medical professional. Readers are advised to consult a physician or other qualified health professional regarding diet and exercise or before acting on any of the information in this book.

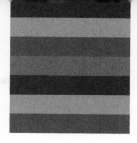

Contents

Part 2

Three Small Steps to Heart-Healthy Living in 5 Weeks

Part 3

Preventing Heart Disease for a Lifetime

Appendices

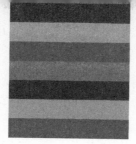

Acknowledgments

We wish to express our gratitude to the countless women we have met at heart screenings, support groups, and community lectures on heart disease. It was their questions, concerns, and frustrations that were the catalyst for this book. These remarkable women provided our inspiration to write *Heart Smart*.

We also wish to thank those who have contributed specifically to this book, for without you, *Heart Smart* would not have come to fruition.

Sincere thanks to our cowriter, Carol Turkington, who was instrumental in helping us with the book proposal. Carol provided us with encouragement and guidance and introduced us to our accomplished and awesome agent, Faith Hamlin, and her terrific assistant, Courtney Miller-Callihan. We could not ask for a better agent than Faith, whose enthusiasm and belief in our passion led us to partner with our wonderful editor, Sheila Curry Oakes. Heartfelt thanks to P.J. Dempsey for her insight, and timely and superb feedback on the manuscript. P.J. always seemed to know when we should be pushed or praised. P.J., we are very grateful to have met you!

Our sincere gratitude to our colleagues in the Division of Cardiology at the North Shore–Long Island Jewish Health System. There are too many to name individually, but Dr. Stacey Rosen, Susan Somerville, Barbara Milone, Jean Lewis, Elizabeth Smith, Karen Falzone, Irene Leff, Tilka Rampersaud, Jaclyn Schindler, Fallon Edwards, Debbie DiMisa, Mary-Ellen Hennessey, and Peter Cafaro; and Drs. Stanley Katz, Stephen Green, Lawrence Ong, Ram Jadonath, and Dennis Dowling are among the best.

Thanks to our friends at the American Heart Association, especially Sue Flor, Kathy Munsch, Darcy Spitz, Michael Weamer, Mark Hurley, Karen Curley, Yamise Fields, Katie Bell, Leslie Holland, Megan Lozito, Julie Del Barto, and Larry Bloustein, for words of encouragement and providing the opportunities to meet many of the women who inspired us to begin writing this book.

Special thanks to those who helped us along our journey: Drs. Michael Palumbo, Sharonne and David Hayes, Donna Polk, Noel Bairey-Merz, Sue Bennett, Jean Cacciabaudo, Michelle Johnson, Allison Spatz, and also Joanne McCarthy,

Hannah Brichter, Edith Katz, Lori and Steve Kany, Barry Shpizner, Lori Russo, Candice Posner, Nancy Loving, and Kathy Kastan.

Heartfelt thanks and love to Connie Burt, who is always generous with her time and willing to share her personal story of heart disease. You are our Heart Smart woman!

We owe tremendous thanks to Darlene Rodriguez for her touching foreword.

Thanks to our colleagues and friends who generously gave of their time to add comments to the book: Drs. Nanatte Wenger, Leslee J. Shaw, Rita Redberg, Martha Gulati, Janet Brill, Robert Bonow, Fay Gary, and Alice Jacobs.

We are truly grateful and honored by the comments of Rehema Ellis, Jane Chesnutt, and the awesome Choose to Move Women: Vernita Morgan and Zulema Esparza.

Thank you is an understatement when it comes to our parents and sisters. Thanks to our parents, Dan and Terry Quinn and Jean Mieres, as well as aunt Barbara Mieres; and to our sisters, Jacqui Leviton, Jacqueline Mieres-Johnston, and Arlene Mieres-Franczak.

Most of all, we wish to thank our husbands, Vincent Parnell and Haskel Fleishaker; and our children, Aubrey and Max Gershenson and Zoë Fleishaker, for their encouragement, understanding, support, and love, without which we would not have been successful in accomplishing our dream.

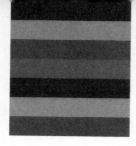

Foreword

*A*s a young Latina growing up in the Bronx, there were so many customs and traditions that I learned as part of my Puerto Rican heritage. We are a passionate, emotional, and fiery people, but loving and affectionate at the same time. There is music and language and a family gathering for every occasion you can possibly think of. And at the center of it all is food. Delicious food that sends a spark through your taste buds and has you salivating as soon as the aroma hits your nose. In a close-knit, poor community, it is the single most sincere way that our grandmothers, mothers, aunts, and neighbors showed their love. And as your friend's mom heaped a mountain of rice, beans, pork chops (fried, of course), and plantains (also fried) onto your plate, you were grateful and she was content, because after all you were way too skinny as far as she was concerned. "*Tu estas muy flaca. . . .* You need to eat."

For many women of color, putting the needs of the family and everyone else before our own needs is what we learned growing up; it's what we watched our mothers do. We do this today in an environment that seems to have more stress, more pressure, more guilt, and less time. An unfortunate by-product of doing this for generations is poor heart health. Many women in our communities are suffering from the effects of obesity, high cholesterol, diabetes, and the number-one killer of us all: heart disease. We fear that getting heart healthy would require us to drastically change what we eat and force us to hit the gym seven days a week, but the wonderful thing about this book is that Jennifer and Terri Ann really get it. They understand the issue from our unique perspective. They will give you tools to make necessary changes without dramatically changing your life, while you get on the road to saving it. They address all of our concerns about giving up all the things that we're used to and they help us step out of our comfort zone without totally giving up our comfort food—the things that remind us of our aunties and *abuelas*.

Heart Smart will help you work on your mind as well as your body, as Jennifer and Terri Ann walk you through small but significant changes, one step at a time. We might not be able to stop putting the needs of others first—and many of us can't change our socioeconomic situation overnight or miraculously erase the stress that comes with it—but what we *can* do is get on the right track today by moving ourselves up higher on that list of priorities. We need to do this so that our daughters, nieces, and granddaughters can follow in our healthy footsteps and not have to deal with heart disease in the staggering numbers that we are dealing with it today. And more important, we need to do this so that we are here, to watch them grow, with a heart that is healthy enough to overflow with love.

—Darlene Rodriguez,
Coanchor, *Today in New York*
WNBC-TV

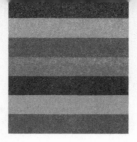

Introduction

$\mathcal{T}$ his book is for all women of Black heritage and Latinas, who are at a higher risk for heart disease than Caucasian women. It is also for all the Latinas and women of Black heritage who are already living with heart disease or one or more risk factors for developing heart disease. It takes just three weeks—twenty-one days—to make a behavior a habit. Good and bad habits are developed by means of two basic factors: reward and repetition. Therefore, our five-week program has a three-step plan for taking charge of your heart and keeping it healthy. Use of this road map will help you on your journey to a heart-healthy life!

When heart disease is mentioned, we almost always think of men as the victims. But heart disease is not just a man's disease. In fact, heart disease kills more women than any other disease, including breast cancer (one in two women in the United States dies of heart disease each year, while one in thirty women dies of breast cancer). Black women (African American, Caribbean American) and Latinas are at the highest risk.

The good news is that great strides have been made in the prevention, early diagnosis, and treatment of heart disease in women. It has taken a long time, but finally the medical community, scientists, and women in general have all increased their awareness of this preventable and treatable disease. It is bittersweet that the problem of heart disease in women has finally made the headlines. Unfortunately, this is because so many millions of women have experienced heart attacks. In fact, the lifetime risk of cardiovascular disease is 25 percent for a forty-year-old woman but increases to almost 50 percent by the time a woman is fifty years old, if she has two risk factors for heart disease. The message is finally being heard and you need to know the facts. It is precisely for this reason that we were inspired to write this book.

Between us, we have more than forty years of medical experience in the field of cardiac medicine, and we know that there is very little information available to Black and Latina women who are at high risk of heart disease or who have had a heart attack. While there are books for women on heart disease, *minority women have their own specific risk factors and lifestyle issues.* Just as heart disease is different in women as compared to men, it also differs when it comes to race. We have written *Heart Smart for Black Women and Latinas* in order to address and answer the questions that have gone unanswered for minority women.

As a Black cardiologist of Trinidadian descent and a cardiac nurse with a passion for educating patients, we have seen firsthand Latinas and Black women with heart disease or risk factors for heart disease who are overwhelmed and frustrated in their attempts to live a heart-healthy life. The complaints and frustrations have all centered around several misperceptions about preventing heart disease, including the myths that women need to change their lifestyles drastically by joining a gym and eating a bland diet, very expensive— and unnecessary—prospects in an attempt to be heart healthy.

We intend to help you understand the science behind heart disease, the simple lifestyle changes that are needed, and the medicines that are available to help you eliminate this potential killer from your life so that you can improve the quality of your daily living and not detract from it.

We don't want you to eliminate your traditional foods; we will teach you how to cook them in a healthier way. We don't want you to go on a starvation diet to lose weight; we will show you how to control your portions and give suggestions for adding exercise to your daily routine. You'll also learn how these minor changes can influence the health of your entire family so that you can finally help break the cycle of heart disease that has become epidemic in our communities. It's also important that you realize that you are not alone. You will see, from the stories of other women, that there are many who are at high risk of heart disease for various reasons, or maybe even in poor health because of actually having suffered a heart attack. You'll have a chance to read their stories and learn from their examples how best to cope with and overcome the medical, cultural, and genetic factors that cause heart disease.

We hope that this book will address your issues and concerns that probably were not covered in other books about women and heart disease. Our experience in the field of cardiology tells us that being diagnosed with heart disease is often accompanied by negativity. The majority of books available to women on heart disease reinforce these negative connotations with titles that include the words "surviving," "coping," and "fighting." But this book is not about the negative; it's about the positive. It's about celebrating life. It is about really living and enjoying a good life. So if you have heart disease, you now have the opportunity to do something about it and get your life back on track. Heart disease is curable, and often those who have had a heart attack and then eliminate the cause are healthier than they ever were before, so let's continue with the good news.

Heart disease is not a death sentence. There are more than eight million women living in the United States who are also victims of heart disease, just like you, but you all have the opportunity to live well and conquer it. In fact, research has shown that women can lower their risk of heart disease by 82 percent simply by making healthy lifestyle changes. A healthy lifestyle change can be as simple as devoting a few minutes a day to moving around. In fact, *any type* of daily exercise or activity is better than being a couch potato. *Any* reduction in calories is better than none, and the addition of *any* new healthier food to your diet is better than eating the same unhealthy food that contributed toward your heart disease. Even if it's only starting with ten minutes of exercise every day, switching to sugar-free drinks, or not eating fried foods, these small changes can make a huge difference.

The point is that you don't have to eliminate *all* of your favorite foods or drastically change the way you live. By taking small steps and slowly decreasing unhealthy habits while slowly substituting healthier habits, you'll not only decrease your risk of heart disease, you'll also feel better.

It's not only what we eat that contributes to heart problems. Stress is also a major factor. Today we understand that the stresses of daily life sometimes get in the way of our making even the smallest changes that can lead to a heart-healthy lifestyle. It's difficult to think about exercising and eating healthy if you're stressed out from work and life at home. We've taken this into account, and our gradual plan will surprise you with its simple suggestions of small changes in your life that you can easily make part of your daily routine. We know our program works because we have seen the proof with our patients. Honestly, we promise that with our five-week program you'll be on your way to living a heart-healthy life—moving more, eating better, living with less stress, and enjoying life more.

This book is for the hundreds of Black women and Latinas we have met over the past five years as patients at community lectures and health screenings. Their questions about how to get heart healthy and their frustrations at not finding information that suited their needs or lifestyles have been the catalyst for this book. They have truly been our source of inspiration.

In working with many women, we have found that there is power in numbers. Although you can follow our program alone, you may want to get a group of your girlfriends together and make this your next book club selection. Having a buddy or two for support and inspiration can keep you on track. It may be the smartest thing you do. You may even save your life or the life of someone you love. Let's get going to a good life!

Jennifer H. Mieres, M.D., F.A.H.A.
Terri Ann Parnell, R.N., M.A.

Part 1

The Double Whammy:
The High Risk of Heart Disease
for Women in General and Black Women
and Latinas in Particular

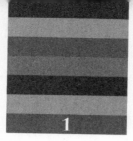

1

Heart Disease: Women's Heart Disease Is Different from Men's

$\mathscr{T}$he lifestyle of most Americans promotes heart disease, and we are a population of "heart attacks waiting to happen." Consider the facts: Cardiovascular disease (which includes heart disease and stroke) is the leading cause of death of American women. In 2004, more than 460,000 women died from cardiovascular disease, compared to 410,000 men. Although most of us fear breast cancer, thanks to the amount of press given this subject, the truth is that women are far more likely to die of heart disease.

Here is a quick look at the numbers: One in eight women will develop breast cancer in her lifetime and one in twenty-six will die of it, but one in three women will die of cardiovascular disease. In fact, a fifty-year-old woman faces a 46 percent risk of developing heart disease and a 31 percent risk of dying from it. Of all the cardiovascular diseases, coronary heart disease, which can lead to a heart attack, and stroke are the number one and three killers of American women.

In this book we focus on reducing your risk of heart disease. By following the steps we outline you will also reduce your risk of a stroke, since many of the same factors that place you at risk for heart disease also increase your chances of having a stroke.

Heart disease and its debilitating effects can be prevented by first recognizing that you are at risk, knowing the signs and the factors that predispose you to heart disease, and then taking simple steps to live a heart-healthy lifestyle.

The Causes of Heart Disease in Women

When it comes to the prevention, diagnosis, and treatment of heart disease, men have traditionally received more attention than women. However, women are at equal risk for heart disease and heart attacks. Although women typically develop heart problems about seven to ten years later in life than men, by about age sixty-five, a woman's risk of heart disease is almost the same as a man's. Blockage of the coronary arteries that supply blood and nutrients to the heart is the leading cause of coronary artery disease and heart attacks in men and women. Certain factors can increase your risk of heart disease. The more risk factors you have, the greater your chance of having a heart attack or stroke. In addition, certain risk factors tend to speed the development of atherosclerosis—the narrowing of arteries due to the buildup of fatty substances. That's why it is important that you identify and eliminate or modify any risk factors you have. Risk factor modification with lifestyle changes as well as taking medication, if needed, can slow the progression of atherosclerosis and help prevent a heart attack.

Although men and women share similar factors that increase their risk of heart disease, such as smoking, high blood pressure (hypertension), diabetes, sedentary lifestyle, high cholesterol, and family history of heart disease, certain factors play a bigger role in the development of heart disease and heart attacks in women. Overall, compared to men, many more women are obese, have a sedentary lifestyle, or have hypertension and diabetes. These particular risk factors play a much more important role in leading to heart disease and heart attacks in women than they do for men.

Why Women of Black and Latino Heritage Have Different Risk Factors From Caucasian Women

The fact that African-American and Hispanic women have as much as a 69 percent higher risk of heart disease than Caucasian women is due in part to their higher incidence of risk factors, including high blood pressure, obesity, physical inactivity, diabetes, and metabolic syndrome. (Metabolic syndrome is a group of risk factors, including abdominal fat, high blood pressure, high cholesterol levels, and insulin resistance or glucose intolerance.) Yet the results of a recent survey indicate that among Black women and Latinas, there is less awareness that being overweight, smoking, physical inactivity, high cholesterol, and a family history of heart disease increase their heart disease risk.

Poor control of cardiovascular risk factors may also account for part of the difference. A recent study published by the American Heart Association found that Black women had higher rates of high blood pressure, diabetes, and high cholesterol than white women. About 56 percent of the Black women in the study had adequate blood pressure control, versus 63 percent of the white women. Furthermore, Black women, despite their higher risk of heart disease, were 10 percent less likely to receive aspirin (to lower the risk of a blood clot, which can block an artery) and 27 percent less likely to receive cholesterol-lowering drugs, known as statins. The results of this study should drive home the fact that women need to be more aware of heart disease risk factors and how to control them. As women, we need to stop underestimating our risk of heart disease.

Color Matters: Why Black Women and Latinas Are at High Risk

Kathleen, a forty-five-year-old African-American woman was referred to me for a stress test because she recently experienced shortness of breath when climbing stairs. At her recent checkup, she was told she was about thirty-five pounds overweight, her blood sugar was elevated, and she was diabetic and needed to start taking medications to control her blood sugar levels. The nurse-practitioner discussed the importance of taking her medications and starting a weight-control program to prevent the horrible complications of diabetes, which include heart disease. This visit was an eye-opener for Kathleen because her father had his first heart attack when he was fifty, and her older brother, who is also diabetic, had heart surgery at age fifty-five. This family history made her determined to change her diet and lifestyle so that she would be around to see her children graduate from high school.

Kathleen and her husband both worked long hours, Kathleen as a legal secretary and he as an elementary school teacher. She reflected on their lifestyle and realized that they were both overweight, he had hypertension, and their diet and family history placed them both at risk for heart disease.

Like Kathleen, most women never dream that they are at risk for heart disease, nor do they have any idea that simply being a woman of color places them at particularly high risk. In fact, one out of every two women of color in the United States will die of heart disease.

Like so many women who experience the early signs of a heart attack or heart disease, Kathleen thought that she was just getting older and her shortness of breath was most likely due to her weight and age. As it turned out, Kathleen's stress test did not show any signs of lack of blood supply to the heart muscle with exercise, but it revealed that her blood pressure was very high during exercise, placing her at risk for heart disease and stroke. Her elevated blood pressure was the cause of her shortness of breath when walking or climbing stairs.

In addition to taking medications for diabetes, Kathleen was started on medication to reduce her blood pressure. She learned that controlling her weight and changing her diet were very important in reducing her risk for heart disease and stroke. Her nurse-practitioner explained the importance of understanding the signs and symptoms of heart disease as well as knowing and controlling her risk for heart disease. Kathleen also learned that by changing her lifestyle, her risk factors for heart disease could be controlled and a heart attack could be prevented. She left the office that day promising herself to change her eating habits as well as lose weight because she did not want to follow in her father's or brother's footsteps.

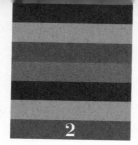

Assessing Your Risk

*I*n order to prevent heart disease and evaluate whether your symptoms are significant, it's important to know what heart disease is, recognize what happens when things go wrong, and have a basic understanding of risk factors.

Heart Disease vs. Heart Attack

You may think that heart disease and heart attack are the same, but they are not. Heart disease includes several different abnormal conditions of the heart and cardiac blood vessels, including coronary artery disease, heart failure, and heart arrhythmias. A heart attack occurs when your arteries have completely closed off and the blood supply can't reach your heart, causing a bit of the muscle to die.

Coronary Artery Disease

Coronary artery disease or coronary heart disease is the most common type of heart disease and involves the coronary arteries—the blood vessels that wrap around the surface of the heart and supply the heart with blood. Fatty deposits called plaque build up inside the walls of these arteries in a process called atherosclerosis (often called "hardening of the arteries"). This buildup narrows the arteries, so that blood has a hard time getting through them to the heart and the heart doesn't get all the blood it needs. Because blood carries oxygen, as the blood level drops, the heart muscle doesn't get enough oxygen. As the blood flow to the heart muscle is reduced and as fatty deposits increase, the blood supply to the heart gets even worse (especially during exercise or emotional stress such as when you are angry or upset). Signs of a poor blood supply to the heart include shortness of breath, chest pain or pressure (doctors call this angina), pain in the left arm or left shoulder, jaw pain, throat pain, heartburn, and general fatigue.

Heart Failure

In heart failure, the heart doesn't actually "fail" and stop working. The heart is unable to effectively pump blood around the body. This poor circulation leads to fluid buildup in the lungs and other body tissues. The symptoms include fatigue, shortness of breath, loss of appetite, nausea, and swelling of the feet and ankles.

Arrhythmia

Arrhythmia is abnormal rate and/or rhythm of the heartbeat—either too low or too high. This can be caused by too little blood reaching the heart, and it reduces the efficiency of the heart, causing too little blood to reach the brain. The symptoms are heart palpitations, light-headedness, shortness of breath, and pain in the chest or neck.

Like Kathleen, it is important that we women know our numbers—blood pressure, blood sugar, cholesterol levels—and determine if our numbers put us at risk.

Risk Factors: How's *Your* Heart?

That's a question we bet you've never been asked! Well, we're reaching out and asking you: What's *your* risk? We suspect most of you don't know. If you're like most women, you probably never knew that one out of five adult women of color has some form of heart disease—right now. Most of *them* have no idea, either.

- As a Black woman, you have almost a 40 percent likelihood of having heart disease and stroke.

- As a Latina, you have a 30 percent chance of having heart disease and stroke.
- Black women and Latinas are more likely than Caucasians to get heart disease because they tend to have more risk factors—obesity, lack of exercise, high blood pressure, and diabetes.
- Women of color are more likely than white women to die from heart disease.

Let's look again at Kathleen, who has diabetes and hypertension. She is now at a very high risk for heart disease—and she is not alone.

- Almost 45 percent of African-American women and 30 percent of Hispanic women have high blood pressure.
- 77 percent of African-American women and 71 percent of Hispanic women in the United States are overweight or obese.

The combination of risk factors in Black women and Latinas places them at the highest risk for heart attacks and stroke.

You are lucky—you are reading this book! Even if you have had a heart attack, you can make small changes to reduce your overall risk.

Are You at Risk for Heart Disease?

Certain risk factors can increase the risk of heart disease. The more risk factors you have, the greater your chance of having a heart attack, because risk factors tend to speed the development of coronary artery disease. Therefore, it is important to identify and eliminate or modify the risk factors, by stopping smoking and with diet, exercise, stress reduction, and sometimes medication, which can slow the progression of heart disease and even help prevent a heart attack. In order to track your progress, you need to make note of your starting point. Just as a physician or nurse writes down information at your first office visit, it is time to start taking notes about yourself. Buy a notebook to devote to your heart health or simply get a blank sheet of paper and start taking your personal health inventory. We will start with your risk.

Risk Factors You Cannot Change

FAMILY HISTORY AND GENETICS

It is said that you can pick your friends, but you can't pick your relatives. This is true for risk of heart disease as well. If you have or had a male first-degree relative (parent or sibling) who had a heart attack or heart disease at age fifty-five or younger or a female first-degree relative who had a heart attack or heart disease at age sixty-five or younger, put them on your risk factor list. A family history of heart disease significantly increases your personal risk. While you can't pick your relatives, once you know about familial risk, you can make different choices because of this increased risk.

Race or ethnicity is also a factor. Black and Hispanic women are generally more likely to have high blood pressure, to smoke, and to be physically inactive, which in turn increase the likelihood of having heart disease.

Like Kathleen, if you have a family history of heart disease—her father had his first heart attack at age fifty—you are at risk. In addition, having siblings with early heart disease—Kathleen's brother had heart disease at age fifty-five—increased her risk. Therefore, discussing your family history of heart disease with your doctor can lead to early identification, proper screening, and treatment for all the risk factors for heart disease, such as high blood pressure, diabetes, high cholesterol, and excess weight. High blood pressure and diabetes begin at an early age in Black and Hispanic women, in some cases as early as the midthirties.

AGE

As we age, our risk for developing heart disease increases. While men over the age of forty-five are also at increased risk, women have about a ten-year lag and become at increased risk for heart disease during the menopause years, generally speaking over the age of fifty-five.

But as we've seen, some of the risk factors such as high blood pressure and diabetes can occur in Black and Hispanic women in their midthirties. Therefore, it is important that you live with heart-healthy habits every day to limit the buildup of fatty plaques in your coronary arteries. This will decrease your risk for heart disease and heart attack as you age.

Risk Factors You Can Change

DIABETES MELLITUS (ELEVATED BLOOD SUGAR)

There are two types of diabetes. Type 1 diabetes develops in childhood or adolescence. With this disease, the pancreas produces no insulin or not enough. It is treated with daily insulin injections. Type 2 diabetes—also called adult-onset diabetes—occurs in adults. Here, the pancreas produces insulin, but the body doesn't use it properly. Insulin allows the body to process sugar. If the body can't do this, blood sugar becomes elevated.

This is a dangerous situation because uncontrolled diabetes can elevate cholesterol levels and can speed up the process of atherosclerosis, which in turn leads to heart disease. Diabetes also has a damaging effect on the arteries in your heart and throughout your body. Your glucose (or blood sugar level) should be 100 mg/dL or less after fasting and 180 mg/dL or less after meals. If you have been told you are a diabetic, add this fact to your personal risk factor list.

Women with diabetes have three to seven times the risk of developing heart disease compared to nondiabetic women. After age forty-five, more women than men develop diabetes. If you control your diabetes with medication, you can decrease your chances of heart disease. In addition, you can help maintain a normal blood sugar by getting regular exercise, changing your eating habits, and controlling your weight.

HYPERTENSION (HIGH BLOOD PRESSURE)

Blood pressure is the measured force of blood against the artery walls and it is recorded as two numbers. The higher number, called the systolic pressure, should be less than 140. The lower number, called the diastolic pressure, should be less than 90. You are diagnosed with hypertension if either number is higher than normal, i.e., 140/90.

It is important to get your blood pressure checked regularly. The recent Women's Take Heart study showed that as many as 60 percent of women with high blood pressure don't know they have it. That is why high blood pressure is called the "silent killer." The American Heart Association estimates that one in four women in the United States has high blood pressure. If you have high blood pressure, your heart, because it is working harder than it should, is subject to excessive wear and tear.

High blood pressure often runs in families and is more often seen in women who are obese and/or eat a diet high in salt. The rate of high blood pressure in Black females age twenty or older is 45 percent and for Hispanic women of the same age it is 30 percent. After age fifty, all women are twice as likely as men to develop high blood pressure. Hypertension is a strong risk factor for heart disease and speeds up the process of atherosclerosis and increases the chances for a heart attack.

Hypertension can be controlled with medication, salt restriction, weight control, and regular exercise. If you have been told you have high blood pressure, add this to your risk factor list.

ABNORMAL CHOLESTEROL LEVELS (HIGH LDL, LOW HDL, HIGH TRIGLYCERIDES)

Cholesterol is a soft, fatlike substance found in the body's cells and circulating in the blood. It can build up with other substances in the lining of the arteries to form a plaque, which narrows the artery and partially blocks blood flow. If a blood clot forms and attaches to the cholesterol plaque, the artery is totally blocked and a heart attack can occur. Thus, a high level of cholesterol accelerates the development of atherosclerosis.

There are two types of cholesterol:

- LDL (low-density lipoprotein) is also known as the "lousy" or "bad" cholesterol. High levels of LDL increase the cholesterol plaque and increase the risk of a heart attack. A diet high in fat and cholesterol is a main cause of high LDL levels.
- HDL (high-density lipoprotein) is the "healthy" or "good" cholesterol. You want higher levels of this cholesterol, which lowers

the risk of heart disease. Prior to menopause, women usually have high levels of HDL. In menopause, LDL cholesterol increases and HDL decreases.

Exercise and food that is low in cholesterol and saturated fats often help decrease the cholesterol levels. In addition, based on the evidence from recent scientific studies, the American Heart Association guidelines for heart disease prevention in women recommend the use of cholesterol-lowering medications, called statins, which have been shown to reduce the incidence of heart disease and heart attack in women. If you have high cholesterol levels, add this risk factor to your list.

Triglyceride is the most common type of fat in the body, and a high triglyceride level is a powerful risk factor for women.

Many women who have heart disease or diabetes have a high level of triglyceride. A high triglyceride level combined with high LDL (bad cholesterol) and low HDL (good cholesterol) seems to speed the buildup of fatty plaque in the coronary arteries.

Recommended Levels of Cholesterol and Triglyceride

LDL cholesterol	Less than 100
HDL cholesterol	Greater than 50
Triglycerides	Less than 150 mg/dL
Total cholesterol	Less than 200 mg/dL

EXCESS BODY WEIGHT (OVERWEIGHT/OBESITY)

Women who are obese have a greater chance of having hypertension, diabetes, and elevated cholesterol levels, all factors that speed the process of atherosclerosis leading to heart disease and heart attacks. In fact, 72 percent of Hispanic women and 77 percent of Black women age twenty or older are obese. Obese women are three times more likely to have heart disease than women with normal body weight for height. If you are obese or overweight, decreasing your weight by as little as ten to twenty pounds will help control your blood pressure, blood sugar, and cholesterol levels, thereby decreasing your overall chance of developing heart disease or having a heart attack.

Although there is no one perfect way to determine whether you are overweight, calculating your body mass index (BMI) serves as the best guide to determine if you are at a heart-healthy weight. A BMI of less than 25 is best. BMI is calculated based on your height and weight. To determine your BMI, locate your height on the table on page 26 and follow it across until you reach a weight that is closest to yours. Then look at the top of the table and you will see your BMI. A BMI of 19 to 24 is considered heart healthy. You are overweight if your BMI is between 25 and 29, and you are obese if your BMI is 30 or greater. Your risk for heart disease increases if your BMI is 25 or greater. Generally speaking, a woman is obese when she is more

Body Mass Index

Body Weight (pounds)

Height (inches)	Normal						Overweight					Obese										Extreme Obesity															
BMI	19	20	21	22	23	24	25	26	27	28	29	30	31	32	33	34	35	36	37	38	39	40	41	42	43	44	45	46	47	48	49	50	51	52	53	54
58	91	96	100	105	110	115	119	124	129	134	138	143	148	153	158	162	167	172	177	181	186	191	196	201	205	210	215	220	224	229	234	239	244	248	253	258
59	94	99	104	109	114	119	124	128	133	138	143	148	153	158	163	168	173	178	183	188	193	198	203	208	212	217	222	227	232	237	242	247	252	257	262	267
60	97	102	107	112	118	123	128	133	138	143	148	153	158	163	168	174	179	184	189	194	199	204	209	215	220	225	230	235	240	245	250	255	261	266	271	276
61	100	106	111	116	122	127	132	137	143	148	153	158	164	169	174	180	185	190	195	201	206	211	217	222	227	232	238	243	248	254	259	264	269	275	280	285
62	104	109	115	120	126	131	136	142	147	153	158	164	169	175	180	186	191	196	202	207	213	218	224	229	235	240	246	251	256	262	267	273	278	284	289	295
63	107	113	118	124	130	135	141	146	152	158	163	169	175	180	186	191	197	203	208	214	220	225	231	237	242	248	254	259	265	270	278	282	287	293	299	304
64	110	116	122	128	134	140	145	151	157	163	169	174	180	186	192	197	204	209	215	221	227	232	238	244	250	256	262	267	273	279	285	291	296	302	308	314
65	114	120	126	132	138	144	150	156	162	168	174	180	186	192	198	204	210	216	222	228	234	240	246	252	258	264	270	276	282	288	294	300	306	312	318	324
66	118	124	130	136	142	148	155	161	167	173	179	186	192	198	204	210	216	223	229	235	241	247	253	260	266	272	278	284	291	297	303	309	315	322	328	334
67	121	127	134	140	146	153	159	166	172	178	185	191	198	204	211	217	223	230	236	242	249	255	261	268	274	280	287	293	299	306	312	319	325	331	338	344
68	125	131	138	144	151	158	164	171	177	184	190	197	203	210	216	223	230	236	243	249	256	262	269	276	282	289	295	302	308	315	322	328	335	341	348	354
69	128	135	142	149	155	162	169	176	182	189	196	203	209	216	223	230	236	243	250	257	263	270	277	284	291	297	304	311	318	324	331	338	345	351	358	365
70	132	139	146	153	160	167	174	181	188	195	202	209	216	222	229	236	243	250	257	264	271	278	285	292	299	306	313	320	327	334	341	348	355	362	369	376
71	136	143	150	157	165	172	179	186	193	200	208	215	222	229	236	243	250	257	265	272	279	286	293	301	308	315	322	329	338	343	351	358	365	372	379	386
72	140	147	154	162	169	177	184	191	199	206	213	221	228	235	242	250	258	265	272	279	287	294	302	309	316	324	331	338	346	353	361	368	375	383	390	397
73	144	151	159	166	174	182	189	197	204	212	219	227	235	242	250	257	265	272	280	288	295	302	310	318	325	333	340	348	355	363	371	378	386	393	401	408
74	148	155	163	171	179	186	194	202	210	218	225	233	241	249	256	264	272	280	287	295	303	311	319	326	334	342	350	358	365	373	381	389	396	404	412	420
75	152	160	168	176	184	192	200	208	216	224	232	240	248	256	264	272	279	287	295	303	311	319	327	335	343	351	359	367	375	383	391	399	407	415	423	431
76	156	164	172	180	189	197	205	213	221	230	238	246	254	263	271	279	287	295	304	312	320	328	336	344	353	361	369	377	385	394	402	410	418	426	435	443

than 30 percent over her ideal body weight based on her height.

As a woman, if you carry most of your weight around the waist and abdomen, you are described as having an apple shape. As fat accumulates around the waist, it increases the risk for heart disease as well as the risk factors of high blood pressure and diabetes. If you have excess fat in your waist or abdominal region, you are at an increased risk for heart disease because abdominal fat is more likely to break down and accumulate in the arteries. A heart-healthy waist size is 35 inches or less. If your waist is larger than 35 inches, add this to your risk factor list.

Being a "little overweight" is like being a "little pregnant!" If you need to shed a few pounds, add this to your risk factor list.

You can maintain an ideal body weight for your height by balancing the number of calories you eat with the number of calories you burn. Start today eating a heart-smart diet. Remember, losing ten to twenty pounds will decrease your risk of heart disease.

CIGARETTE SMOKING AND EXPOSURE TO SECONDHAND SMOKE

If you smoke, you are at an increased risk for a heart attack. There are no ifs, ands, or buts about it. According to the American Heart Association, smoking is the leading preventable cause of heart disease in women. Almost 11 percent of Hispanic women and 18 percent of Black women eighteen years and older smoke. In general, women smokers are six times more likely to have coronary artery disease than nonsmokers. Smoking has a negative impact on cholesterol levels and may also encourage blood platelets to clump together in a coronary artery, making it more likely that a heart attack will occur. As few as five cigarettes a day can double the risk for coronary artery disease. The good news is that when a woman stops smoking, her risk of heart disease immediately starts to drop, and over time her risk will become about the same as if she never smoked.

We aren't going to lecture you about all the other horrible health effects of smoking. If you smoke, even "a little," add it to your risk factor list and then walk over to your cigarettes and say good-bye as you toss them in the trash! Do this and take the first step in making yourself healthier.

However, we realize it is not easy to quit smoking cold turkey. Luckily there are new medications, including patches, gum, and pills, that your doctor can prescribe to help you quit. So if you smoke, schedule a visit with your doctor to discuss the best way to stop.

You can also get help in becoming smoke-free by calling the National Cancer Institute's Smoking Quitline, 1-877-44U-Quit. They have trained personnel who can give advice on how you can begin the process of quitting.

Exposure to secondhand smoke also increases your risk of heart disease. Banish friends and family members to the outdoors to smoke (if you can't persuade them to quit along with you) and sit in no-smoking public areas.

When you quit, let us be the first to offer you congratulations! Now take a pretty basket or a jar and place it where you used to keep your cigarettes at home. Each time you want to buy a pack of cigarettes, place the money you would have spent on the cigarettes in the basket. In no time at all, you will have a "basket of money" to use for healthier habits and treats, or perhaps a short vacation. If you continue to smoke, make a note of this for your list of risk factors.

INACTIVE LIFESTYLE (PHYSICAL INACTIVITY)

An inactive lifestyle leads to a higher incidence of hypertension, obesity, and elevated cholesterol levels. Women who are physically active have a 50 percent decrease in the incidence of heart disease.

Black and Hispanic women tend to be less active than Caucasian women. Of Black women age eighteen and older, 55 percent are inactive, compared to 36 percent of white women. Almost 40 percent of Hispanic women age eighteen and older are physically inactive.

You do not need to join a gym. Just taking a brisk walk for thirty minutes a day and using the stairs instead of the elevator will give you all the workout you need. By the way, three brisk ten-minute walks have the same heart benefit as one uninterrupted thirty-minute workout.

Thirty to forty-five minutes of moderate aerobic exercise (walking, dancing, bicycling, or housework) three times a week can decrease your chances for heart disease and help control your blood pressure, blood sugar, and cholesterol. If you have an inactive lifestyle in general, add this to your personal risk factor list.

STRESS (HECTIC LIFESTYLE)

We all experience stress sometimes. But the important aspect of stress in terms of heart health is the amount we feel and the way we react to it. How you react to stress is called the stress response. Responses to stress are different in each of us. What one woman considers a stressful situation might be no big deal to another. More and more research is being done on the relationship of stress to the risk of heart disease. Stress certainly affects heart disease, but what is not known is if stress in and of itself acts as an isolated or independent risk factor. Stress impacts the other previously mentioned risk factors of heart disease such as high blood pressure, obesity, cholesterol levels, smoking, and physical inactivity.

Take a look at your daily routine, including your personal, family, and working relationships, and think about whether you have a "stressful routine" in general. Do you have any time for just you? Are you ever the priority on your to-do list? Do you feel refreshed at the end of your weekend, ready to tackle the new week? Managing stress is important for overall health as well as your heart health!

If you feel stressed regularly, add this to your personal risk factor list.

New Guidelines for Prevention of Heart Disease in Women

The first scientifically based guidelines about heart disease prevention were published in February 2004 and updated in 2007 by the American Heart Association. The important highlights are:

- Heart disease can be prevented or controlled with changes in lifestyle and the use of medications to control your risk factors. Lifestyle changes are the most important in preventing heart disease.
- Awareness, knowledge, and action are by far the most important factors in saying good-bye to the number one killer of women.

Assessing Your Risk Factors

Review your list of risk factors before you take the following quiz.

RISK FACTOR QUIZ

We included the common risk factors of heart disease in this simple quiz. After honestly answering these questions, you'll know what your personal heart disease risk really is. Circle yes or no—it's as simple as that.

Risk Factors You Can't Control

1. Gender

I am Black or Latina   Yes   No

2. Your Medical History

I have been postmenopausal for at least seven years.   Yes   No

I have had a total hysterectomy and my ovaries were removed.   Yes   No

I have coronary heart disease or angina (chest pain).   Yes   No

I have already had a heart attack.   Yes   No

I have had a stroke, ministroke, or TIA

(transient ischemic attack).   Yes   No

I have disease or blockages in the arteries of my legs.   Yes   No

3. Family Medical History and Age

I have or had a father or brother who had coronary heart

disease before age fifty-five.   Yes   No

I have or had a mother or sister who had coronary heart

disease before age sixty-five.   Yes   No

I am older than fifty-five.   Yes   No

Risk Factors That You Can Change

4. Diabetes

I've been told I have diabetes or I am being treated

for diabetes.   Yes   No

My fasting (no food for several hours before the blood test)

blood sugar is 100 mg/dL or higher.   Yes   No

My blood sugar without fasting is 180 mg/dL or higher.   Yes   No

5. Cholesterol

My total cholesterol is 200 mg/dL or higher.   Yes   No

My HDL (good cholesterol) level is less than 50 mg/dL.   Yes   No

My LDL (bad cholesterol) is greater than 100 mg/dL.   Yes   No

6. High Blood Pressure

I am being treated for high blood pressure.   Yes   No

My blood pressure on two or more readings has been

higher than 120/80.   Yes   No

7. Weight

I have a BMI (body mass index) of 25 or higher.

(A BMI of 25 to 29.9 = overweight,

a BMI of 30 or higher = obese.)   Yes   No

My waist measurement is more than 35 inches.   Yes   No

Contributing Risk Factors

8. Cigarette Smoking

I smoke cigarettes.   Yes   No

I live or work with people who smoke cigarettes in

my presence.   Yes   No

9. Daily Physical Activity

I get less than thirty minutes a day of physical activity

on most days of the week.   Yes   No

10. Stress

I feel like I am under stress most of the time.	Yes No

I am always on the go, doing for everyone else, and never

take any time for myself to regroup and recharge.	Yes No
Lately I have an overwhelming sense of doom and gloom.	Yes No

Know Your Score

How many times did you circle yes? Obviously, the more yeses, the higher your risk for heart disease. Not all risk factors are equal. Smoking, for example, is much more dangerous than slightly elevated blood pressure (though even a small increase in blood pressure needs to be treated). Whether you circled yes only once or every single time, please finish reading this book. Then try to make the recommended lifestyle changes. If you haven't seen your doctor recently, make an appointment—and bring this checklist with you. Finally, if you couldn't answer some of the questions because you have no idea what your blood pressure and cholesterol readings (and blood sugar if you are diabetic) are, you should see your doctor right now and get tested.

You may be asking, "Why should I make any changes at all? I feel fine!" And that's the problem with heart disease—most of us have no idea of our true health risks in the early stages, when we really could do something about making ourselves healthier.

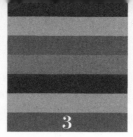

3

Don't Be a Statistic: It's Never Too Late to Get on the Road to Heart Health

$\mathcal{B}$eatrice lay on the examining table as the sedative dripped into her vein, the harsh lights fading as she drifted in and out of a twilight state. Heart disease! She couldn't believe it. One year ago she'd been diagnosed with high blood pressure, but she'd thought that she had been doing pretty well on medication, although her blood pressure was still elevated on her last visit to the doctor. Her doctor increased her dosage of blood pressure medication and reminded her that if she lost weight, her medications might be able to be reduced. Beatrice knew she was twenty pounds overweight, but she'd been exercising off and on without much success, and she didn't want to give up her favorite fried chicken, cakes, and pies. She put off thinking about her high blood pressure and weight problems until the day before her foot surgery, when her doctor discovered that her electrocardiogram (EKG) was abnormal. When questioned by the doctor, Beatrice admitted that for the past month she had noticed shortness of breath and heartburn while performing her regular household chores. Beatrice was sent for a stress test later that day, which showed that one of her arteries was almost completely blocked. Unable to get enough blood when she was performing exercise or strenuous activities, her heart was slowly starving to death.

Beatrice is one of the lucky ones. She was diagnosed and treated before any permanent damage to her heart had occurred. Shocked into awareness, she began her road to a healthier heart by starting on a five-week plan to heart health featuring small daily changes toward a healthier lifestyle. First she started walking up two flights of stairs at work instead of taking the elevator. She took a five-minute walk around the office during her lunch hour, and she and her husband began to walk around the block after dinner at least three nights a week. She slowly began to work on her diet too. First, she added a new fruit or vegetable serving to her diet each day, removing one serving of sweets or fried food. She began roasting meat instead of frying it and made sure that her fridge was filled with heart-healthy snacks so there was no temptation. She also began to schedule time into her day to de-stress on her lunch hour while at work, quietly listening to music or reading a book. After five weeks on this plan, her blood pressure and cholesterol were significantly lower, she had lost eight pounds, and she felt encouraged and had more energy.

Recent guidelines for women from the American Heart Association clearly state that once coronary artery disease is evident, women need to be aggressively managed to reduce complications and death from heart attacks. Having had a 90 percent blockage of a coronary artery, and having the blockage opened by having a stent inserted, was the first step for Beatrice. She also needed to get her bad cholesterol (LDL) down to 70, needed to take an aspirin a day, "get moving" regularly, and keep her blood pressure below 120/80.

Leading a Healthy Lifestyle: It Is All About Prevention!

Prevention pays. One year later, Beatrice continues her simple three-step approach to preventing more heart disease. She has kept notes on her heart-healthy lifestyle, records her daily activities, and keeps a record of her heart-healthy numbers: total cholesterol below 200 and LDL (bad cholesterol) below 100, blood sugar below 100, and a BMI of 24. She is eating a heart-healthy diet, she walks at least thirty minutes four days a week, and she finds some quiet time for stress reduction. She has lost more than twenty pounds and has been able to maintain this heart-healthy body weight. Her small steps have resulted in big gains in her wish to conquer heart disease.

As she read more about heart disease and realized that

it could be prevented, she reflected on what she could have done differently. She learned that as an African-American woman, she was at a much higher risk of heart disease and that her high blood pressure increased her chances of having a heart attack. She regrets that she did not pay closer attention to controlling her blood pressure.

Following a heart-healthy lifestyle is simple. It does not mean that you must deprive yourself of your favorite foods. Instead, by finding ways to incorporate heart-healthy habits into your lifestyle, you will be well on your way to enjoying a healthier life for years to come.

If you have any of the risk factors for heart disease—smoking, high blood pressure, high cholesterol, diabetes, sedentary lifestyle, or being overweight—it is important that you speak to your doctor or nurse-practitioner about reducing your risk for heart disease.

The most recent American Heart Association guidelines for prevention of heart disease in women recommend that women should be more aggressively managed to prevent heart disease, beginning with earlier diagnosis and careful evaluation of risk factors. Knowing if you have any symptoms is the best way to start, because many can be subtle. Remember, though, that just looking for symptoms is not a substitute for your regular medical checkup. Heart disease is a silent killer. Just as checking for a lump in your breast doesn't substitute for a mammogram, calculating potential symptoms is no substitute for a thorough checkup with your health-care practitioner. Some risk factors you just cannot see or feel.

Recognizing Cardiac Symptoms

Knowing your risk and the signs of a heart attack is very powerful. Use this information to your advantage.

Beatrice failed to recognize that her shortness of breath and heartburn when she did her household chores were signs of heart disease and in fact was a cry for more blood supply to her heart. Recognizing the signs of heart disease is something of a challenge for women. Doctors tend to look for the most common symptom (in men and women): chest pain or discomfort. Often they fail to pay attention to symptoms more common to women than men: shortness of breath, heartburn, nausea and vomiting, and back or jaw pain. The presence of atypical signs delayed Beatrice's visit to the doctor as she did not think of heart disease as a cause of her symptoms.

The most common or classic signs of heart attack in women are:

- uncomfortable pressure, fullness, squeezing, or pain in the center of the chest that lasts more than a few minutes, or goes away and then comes back
- pain that begins in the chest and spreads to the shoulders, neck, jaw, or arms

- chest discomfort accompanied by sweating, nausea, light-headness, fainting, or shortness of breath

Don't ignore the less common or atypical symptoms of heart attack and heart disease:

- nausea, dizziness, shortness of breath or difficulty breathing, weakness or fatigue, stomach or abdominal pain, palpitations, cold sweats, paleness
- unexplained anxiety and an overwhelming feeling of "doom and gloom"

Although Beatrice did not have a heart attack, she was at a very high risk of having a completely blocked coronary artery, which could lead to a heart attack. She now knew that she was not merely "at risk" for coronary disease but that she actually had coronary disease and was lucky to have been treated before she suffered a heart attack.

Overcome Genetics and Lifestyle to Reduce Heart Disease

Consider having a heart disease discussion with your doctor and together figure out your personal risk for heart disease. Your doctor is your ally. Be honest about your lifestyle and behaviors. Take your medications for high blood pressure, cholesterol-lowering medication, and/or diabetes medications. Realize that you can greatly improve your outcomes by incorporating heart-healthy habits into your lifestyle. Heart-healthy habits add to the effects of medications in controlling your risk factors for heart disease. And, by modifying your eating and losing weight, you may be able to decrease your medications. Warning: Don't stop taking or take less of your medications just because you "feel better." Talk to your doctor.

Healthy Lifestyle Changes

Taking action to be heart healthy is easier than you may think. Start by choosing one or two lifestyle habits that are easiest for you to change. Changing your diet to cut back on fried foods, sweet pastries, and fatty desserts, increasing your servings of fruits and vegetables, and eating fish twice a week, will get you on your way to conquering heart disease. Prepare healthy snacks to have on hand at home, at the office, and on the road. Cut back on your serving sizes of meat—one serving should be the size of a deck of cards or the palm of your hand. Become more active and make an attempt to eventually incorporate up to thirty minutes of activity in your daily routine.

Beatrice increased her daily activity by getting off the bus two stops early and walking for ten minutes the rest of the way to work. She did this most days of the week, even when there was mild rain or snow. It actually made her feel better to have been active at the start of her day and helped set the tone for the rest of her day. She thought twice when her coworker offered her a doughnut in the morning and chose not to eat the sweet. It was hard to ruin what she already did for the day!

Small steps can result in big gains in the fight against heart disease. If you've been diagnosed with even one risk factor, it is important that you get advice from your doctor and take any medications he or she prescribes. Getting regular checkups is the only way to identify early signs of heart disease. See your doctor annually (or more often if your doctor recommends). Use your birthday as a reminder to schedule an appointment. It may be the best gift you can give yourself! By discussing all your heart disease symptoms with your doctor, you will be taking the first step in acknowledging heart disease. It's a good thing to know your risk, as knowledge is power. Use it to your advantage by seeking quick treatment, even if it means going to the emergency room if you are having signs of a heart attack—that could prevent or limit a full-blown attack.

Now is your chance to be healthier than you've ever been before. By paying attention to the risk factors and partnering with your doctor to eliminate or control those risks—quitting smoking, losing weight, managing stress, and so on—you will be well on the road to avoiding heart disease.

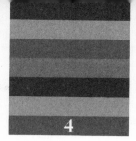

Listen to Your Body

*M*aria is a forty-nine-year-old Hispanic woman who was quite active, primarily caring for her two children and working part-time at a local bank. Her daily routine included walking about a quarter of a mile from the train station to her job. However, she began to notice that her energy level was decreasing and that she experienced fatigue after walking the short distance to work. In addition, on weekends she noted that while doing the grocery shopping, she was tired after pushing the grocery cart around the store and she began parking her car next to the entrance.

At first Maria assumed that she was tired because she was getting older and had recently entered menopause. However, her lack of energy level and easy fatigue continued for about five months, until it was time for her annual checkup. She described her diminishing energy to her doctor. Based on blood tests run at the visit, her doctor told her that her cholesterol was okay, and since she did not have a family history of heart disease, the symptoms were not likely to be related to her heart. However, because this was the second time that her blood pressure was elevated, her doctor decided that she should undergo a treadmill exercise stress test to see if elevated blood pressure with exercise was the cause of her fatigue and decrease in energy.

Maria was able to exercise on the treadmill in her doctor's office for only four minutes, and the test was stopped due to fatigue and very elevated blood pressure. She was placed on medications to control her blood pressure and was told that if she could lose fifteen pounds her blood pressure might be better controlled.

Two months later, I met Maria in the emergency room. That morning at work, her fatigue was accompanied by severe shortness of breath and she felt sweaty. She noticed mild chest discomfort. Her coworkers called an ambulance and when she arrived at the emergency room, it was clear from an electrocardiogram (EKG) that she was having a heart attack. An angiogram (a kind of X-ray) several hours later revealed that one of the arteries that supplied her heart had a significant blockage. At age forty-nine, Maria had a stent placed in the artery to keep it open and increase the blood flow to her heart.

It was fortunate that Maria came to the emergency room right away because it was less than three hours from the onset of her first symptoms until her vessel was opened with the stent. The sooner you get treatment, the better.

As Maria reflected on the three months prior to her heart attack, she realized that her high blood pressure, which was not well controlled, placed her at increased risk for heart disease. Her decrease in exercise ability and her feeling of fatigue with walking were signs that her heart was not getting enough blood, a signal that she had heart disease. A signal that she ignored.

Pay Attention to a Change in Exercise Ability

If you exercise regularly or are very active, you are at a lower risk of heart attack and stroke. Therefore, it is very important that you keep track of changes in your exercise ability, such as becoming fatigued sooner than usual with walking or any other activity. This may indicate heart disease. Many women do not get the same warning signs of heart disease as men, and studies have shown that a change in exercise capacity can be a marker of heart disease in women, especially in Black women and Latinas. Monitoring your ability to exercise provides a way to gauge whether you may be developing heart disease. Even minor changes in your heart function can make you consciously or unconsciously exercise less vigorously. You may tell yourself that you've been stressed at work or the cold weather has kept you indoors and you think you're just out of shape—check in with your doctor anyway. When you do go to the doctor, don't minimize how you are feeling. Tell it like it is and let the doctor decide if it is nothing after all— or if it is something.

Know What You Need to Change

Before leaving the hospital, Maria discussed her new heart-healthy plan with the nurse-practitioner. Together they focused on three important changes she needed to implement to help prevent another heart attack.

1. **Eat healthy.** Maria promised to eat more colorful fruits and vegetables and less fried foods, eliminate sugary sodas, eat baked or broiled fish at least twice a week, and add more legumes and beans.
2. **Get moving.** Maria decided to schedule a playdate with her two children once a week: walk to the park and get in some physical activity, throw a ball around, or ride bicycles together. She was also going to try to walk for ten minutes at least four days a week. This would be much more than she was currently doing. Her only exercise now was walking from the train to the bank where she worked.
3. **Stress less.** Maria agreed to try to put herself at the top of her list one to two times a week as a start. When she was younger, she enjoyed salsa dancing—she was going to give a

girlfriend a call and ask if she would like to go dancing every two weeks. Just the thought of dancing again brought a smile to Maria's face.

The Good Stuff You'll Notice

Here's what Maria found after a few weeks:

- When her children came home from school, they could take one look at her and know whether or not she exercised that day. They said they could tell by the way she spoke to them, her facial expressions, and her entire mood. She was more relaxed and had a positive outlook on the days she took time for herself and exercised a bit.
- She had more energy. She didn't feel exhausted at the end of the day. She didn't feel like life was an endurance contest anymore, either.
- Because she was less tired, she felt that her memory was sharper and she was more interested in day-to-day things.

Putting it plainly, Maria was enjoying life more and had a better outlook about everything on most days.

Don't Be Afraid to Change—Especially Making Positive Changes

Dealing with change can be very hard for many women, especially when it has to do with habits that tie us to our families, our traditions, and our culture. You can increase the likelihood of succeeding with the change by focusing your attention on the outcome of the change. For example, if you look ahead and can see yourself in better shape, playing with your grandchild, or attending your son's high school graduation, it helps you to stick to the changes. You will be seeing the glass half full instead of half empty.

Many times we feel stressed about making a change because we feel that we have no choice or that we are out of control or do not know the outcome of the change. If you had to change because you were being given a brand-new car or a large luxurious home, or you just won the lottery, you would feel much more positive about that type of change. So focus on the positive.

You can control your thoughts, so be optimistic and consider yourself lucky or blessed that you have this opportunity to make changes. Not all women are so lucky. How you feel about the changes you are about to make is the most important factor in determining the result. Think positive thoughts for positive changes, and you are on your way to a heart-healthy lifestyle!

An easy way to make changes is to take them on slowly, step by step, so that you are not overwhelmed. The five-week program will help you prepare for and implement positive changes in your life and will give you the tools to maintain these changes so you stay heart healthy for life.

Understanding the 5-Week
Heart-Smart Program

Week One involves getting ready and cleaning out. Preparing yourself for change will help make you successful and less stressed. The more prepared you are, the less likely you are to stumble.

Week Two focuses on getting moving!—what you can do, how to do it, whom to do it with, and how to include the family (if you would like). We've provided helpful hints on how not to sabotage yourself before you get started and how to increase your activity without much change to your lifestyle.

Week Three adds heart-healthy eating to your life. We offer suggestions for small gradual changes such as adding one fruit or vegetable a day or substituting one healthier food item for a poor quality one. You will find tips about portion control and how to quickly assess correct portions. We suggest substitutions for traditional dishes, so that you can still enjoy your favorite cultural foods, and give you ideas for food shopping and eating out.

Week Four discusses ways to decrease the stress in your life and how to change the way you react to it if you cannot avoid it.

Week Five puts it all together by using the acronym FEAST:

Family and friends
Eat healthy
Active lifestyle
Stress reduction
Take control of your life!

So let's get going. In just five weeks you will be a heart-smart woman.

Part 2

Three Small Steps to Heart-Healthy

Living in 5 Weeks

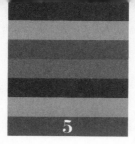

Week One: Get Ready by "Setting the Table" for the Rest of Your Life!

*I*t's now time to start the five-week program to better heart health. The program consists of three small steps you will need to integrate into your life:

- Step 1: Get moving
- Step 2: Eat healthier
- Step 3: Lessen the stress

But first you'll have to prepare yourself mentally and physically before you get down to the business of living a heart-healthy life! We hope you'll be surprised when you see how easy it is to make these three steps part of your life and how quickly you notice improvements in your appearance and attitude. So let's jump in, starting with preparing to eat healthy, because although good food choices keep you in tip-top health, bad food choices contribute to the primary reason we have heart disease in the first place: obesity. Overweight and obesity in turn lead to or complicate diabetes, high blood pressure, and high cholesterol—all contributors to heart disease.

The first thing you need to do is to get your pantry and refrigerator cleaned out and restocked with the foods that will start you on your healthy lifestyle.

Refrigerator Purge

Take a good look inside your fridge. What's in there? We're betting that you have whole milk, butter, lard, ketchup, and salad dressing (which can be loaded with sugar), fruit nectars, sugary sodas, some leftovers (probably some cold fried chicken, pot roast, fried rice, and a dessert or two). Don't forget the freezer. Do you have ice cream, popsicles, frozen pizzas, frozen waffles, TV dinners, and more? These are the foods that you are going to get rid of either by tossing them out or giving them away to friends or a nearby soup kitchen or shelter. (Just because these foods don't fit into your new eating style doesn't mean that others can't eat them.) Any food that is high in fat, bad carbohydrates, and sugar has no place in your new life. We are going to focus on healthy foods that you'll enjoy and that will keep you satisfied so that you don't miss the stuff you used to eat.

A word about carbs. Good carbohydrates metabolize slowly, releasing glucose gradually into the bloodstream. (This is especially important if you are diabetic.) In general, think brown—whole-grain bread, brown rice, whole wheat pasta, yams. Fresh fruits and vegetables are full of good carbs.

Heart-Healthy Foods
Dairy Products

You are now going to choose only low-fat or fat-free dairy products or soy products, which are also low in fat, salt, and sugar. There are lots of choices of low-fat dairy products. If you've never noticed, you'll be in for a pleasant surprise the next time you go to the supermarket. For example, there are all kinds of low-fat cheeses available prepackaged in the dairy case or in the deli part of the supermarket. In fact, many manufacturers of name-brand quality cheese products also make low-fat alternatives that taste surprisingly similar to their full-fat counterparts.

Likewise, there is no need to think of skim milk as the watered-down or gray-colored milk of the past. The newest skim products look and taste (and cook) like whole milk. There are other milk choices as well—soy and rice milk are tastier to some than skim milk. You can even find nonfat half-and-half for your coffee and nonfat or low-fat cream cheese.

For the most part, though, we're sticking to the low-fat varieties because they taste better than nonfat, except for milk and yogurt. Healthy changes won't make you feel deprived. It may take a few purchases to find the brand and type that you and your family prefer, but it is worth the investment of time in the long run!

Egg substitutes aren't really substitutes; they are egg whites that have been made to look like whole eggs. You really can't tell the difference in eating or baking. Or you can buy regular eggs and just use the whites—there is no added effort or cost this way.

Dairy Choices

- low-fat, nonfat or soy yogurt
- low-fat cottage cheese
- reduced-fat or part-skim cheese
- low-fat or nonfat sour cream
- skim or 1% milk (or soy or rice milk if you are lactose intolerant)
- no-sugar-added, low-fat ice cream, low-fat frozen yogurt, or soy ice cream
- butter spreads (like Healthy Balance, Soy Garden)
- eggs (whole and packaged) or cartons of egg whites or Egg Beaters

Meat and Fish

Protein is an important nutrient, so leave room in the freezer to stock healthy meats and fish. You'll probably find that you'll have to make your portions smaller, but you won't be eliminating meat or fish from your life. Use your head when buying healthier cuts of meat, which means staying away from fatty pork bacon, ribs, big fatty steaks, and chuck roasts. Always buy the leaner cuts of beef. If you are not sure, ask the butcher or person in the meat department of the supermarket for help.

Meat, Poultry, and Fish Choices

- lean red meat (top or bottom round)
- ground meat (no more than 20% fat)
- chicken (fresh or frozen, not precooked)—buy skinless or remove the skin before cooking rather than fried chicken patties; white meat has fewer calories than dark
- chicken sausage (many varieties are available)
- turkey (parts and ground)
- turkey bacon and turkey sausage, both Italian-style and breakfast-style links
- lean pork (boneless chops are great)
- pork tenderloin
- any plain unprocessed fish or shellfish (not fish sticks or frozen fried fish)—cod, tuna, and halibut are lower in total fat than many meat and poultry products; salmon, mackerel, and herring

are cold-water fish that are rich sources of omega-3 fats, which help lower your triglycerides (blood fats)

Beverages

Anything with sugar is out. Ditch the full-sugar sodas and cut down on the fruit nectars and fruit juices (you should be eating fresh fruit, anyway, but we're getting ahead of ourselves). The beverage aisle is loaded with many fruit-flavored no-calorie or very low-calorie waters these days, so buy a few different kinds until you find a favorite.

Beverage Choices
- diet sodas (caffeine free is best)
- low-sugar natural fruit juices—not fruit mixes
- fruit nectars (only if you mix them with club soda)
- iced tea (unsweetened or artificially sweetened, or make your own)
- flavored waters
- green tea

Produce

Fresh and frozen fruits and vegetables are great healthy choices. If you must use canned products, choose only low-sodium canned vegetables and canned fruit packed in its natural juices or water. Keep your fridge full of fresh vegetables for cooking and snacking, and try to have fresh fruits to add to your breakfast or for desserts and snacking. Choose any you like—there are no horribly bad choices when it comes to fresh produce. Here are some suggestions of those that can double as snacks.

Produce Choices

- apples
- bananas
- berries—especially blueberries, strawberries, raspberries
- breadfruit
- cherries
- chironja (an orange-grapefruit hybrid)
- grapes—can be frozen for a refreshing snack
- guavas
- mamey (a tropical melon)
- mangoes
- melon chunks
- oranges
- peaches
- pears
- pineapple chunks
- plums
- broccoli and cauliflower florets—dip in salsa
- carrots
- celery
- radishes
- sweet peppers—red, yellow, and green

Condiments

Staples such as ketchup (high in sugar) and mayonnaise (high in fat) are in everyone's fridge, but you can switch to low-fat varieties, especially when you are going to use large amounts, such as when making potato salad or baked beans (but even then, use less than you used to). Switch to mustards, oil and vinegar, or low-fat salad dressings whenever possible, as they are much healthier.

Condiment Choices
- ketchup
- low-fat mayonnaise
- low-fat salad dressings (or stick to homemade vinegar-and-oil dressings, which are the best choice)
- low- or no-sugar fruit spreads
- pickles
- mustard
- salsa—great on chicken, fish, potatoes, and eggs, and in salads

Purging the Pantry

Now, as you did in the refrigerator, take a good look at what you've accumulated over the years (yes, years—chances are, if you're like most of us, you'll find some packages of food that are older than your children). Get two empty boxes. Mark one box "garbage," for the foods with expired dates you never got around to making, or foods no one in your family likes. The other box is for food to donate or give away: potato chips, regular pretzels, taco chips (chips of any kind), packaged cookies, cakes, pies, cake mixes, full-fat baking mixes, nuts processed in oil, etc. If in doubt, check the list of ingredients. If sugar or fat is one of the first three ingredients, get it out of your house. If your pantry is looking bare, here's what you need to give it a healthy makeover:

Snacks
- 100% whole-grain or wheat pretzels
- raw, unsalted almonds or cashews
- 100% whole-grain or 100% whole wheat breads
- plain graham crackers
- whole-grain baked crackers
- high-fiber cereals (5 or more grams of fiber per serving)

Staples
- unbleached flour
- whole wheat flour
- sugar substitute (such as Splenda granular that can also be used in baking)
- coffee
- tea
- low-sodium soups and broths
- canned fish (salmon, tuna, herring, sardines) packed only in water or tomato sauce
- healthy oils (olive, canola, safflower)

- beans and lentils
- brown rice or brown rice blends
- oatmeal
- spaghetti sauce (low sodium, low sugar)
- whole wheat pasta
- low-salt canned vegetables
- cornmeal
- canned tomatoes, whole and diced
- almond butter

These are by no means complete lists, but they will get you started and make you aware of the types of foods you should have at your fingertips so that you are always able to create a healthy meal.

Shopping Tips
Shop the Walls

Whenever you go food shopping, "shop the walls." If you stick to the perimeter of the grocery store to do most your shopping, you won't be tempted by the high-sugar, high-fat snacks and foods. Produce, meats, fish, dairy, and deli products are sold along each of the three sides of a supermarket. If you need to go through the bakery to get from the deli to the fish, well, pick up some whole-grain bread on the way.

Make a Master Shopping List

This is the list you'll use every time you go shopping to help you save time and avoid unhealthy impulse purchases. Divide the list into categories, leaving enough room to list the foods you need. If you have a computer, make a template so it's ready to print out and fill in every week or month, or write it by hand and photocopy it so you always have a blank shopping list ready to fill out before every trip to the supermarket.

Our suggestion is to list your categories in the order in which the foods are arranged in your local market. For example, Karen has to walk through the produce department when she enters the store, which leads to the deli and then to the meat and fish department. (Remember, walk the walls first for staples.) After you get these categories down, then list the ones in the middle of the store and go to only those sections in those aisles. Don't give in to browsing because you will be tempted by high-fat, high-sugar foods you are trying to avoid, and before you know it you'll have replaced all the stuff you threw away. A list will help you not to forget anything and waste time having to go back for items you forgot. Getting your new shopping system down will take time at first, but it is worth it in the long run. Keep the list out in plain sight, and add to it as you use up staples or someone asks for something special. By the time you are ready to go shopping, your list will be filled in with many items and will save you time.

Never Shop When You're Hungry

We guarantee that you will not stick to your shopping list if you shop when you're hungry. Do your food shopping after dinner or after breakfast or lunch—never before—and buy only what is on your list.

Shop for the Month

Now that you've cleaned out the pantry and know which foods are healthy choices, get the family involved and start actually planning what you're going to eat for the month. If that is too big of an expense for you, then plan at least a week in advance. The idea is to educate yourself so that you develop your own system of thinking and planning what you'd like to eat and then shop for the healthy ingredients for those meals. If you stock up, you'll always have groceries on hand, and you will be less likely to run out for fast food.

Get Family or Friends Involved

Your family is going to be eating the same foods as you (granted, you will probably get some occasional sugary snacks or cereals for the kids, but limit these so that you can teach them early about good eating habits). If you have a shopping list you will actually stick to, then you can send your older children off to get specific items. If you live alone, get together with a girlfriend, sister, niece, or other relative and do your shopping together. Having company will make the whole trip go faster and get you home sooner so that you can start on your other healthy activities. (And you are less likely to buy a gallon of ice cream if there is a witness!)

Share the Load

To make shopping and cooking more fun, assign a day of the week for each member in your household to cook or, if they are too young to cook or you don't want them any-where near your kitchen, let each person choose the menu for a specific day. For example, Monday can be your son's Italian day, Tuesday can be your choice of vegetarian, and Wednesday can be Popi's choice, Mexican. This encourages involvement and educates family members to the rules of good eating and empowers them to create or have you serve food they actually want to eat. Come up with your own ideas to keep your family involved—and get the bonus of having a family meal together.

If you live alone, you can buddy up with a few girl-friends or relatives and cook for each other. In this case, the choice of meal is up to the cook. As an alternative, each of you can make one meal and package and freeze it for each member of your group. Set one day to exchange these pre-portioned meals, and that way you will each have four meals in your freezer that are perfect for your heart-healthy lifestyle.

Create a Special Meal Planner

Get a loose-leaf binder and divide it into categories by meals—breakfast, lunch, dinner, and snacks or desserts. As you try new recipes, you can file them in the correct section and write comments such as "José really liked this," "Quick and easy to make," and so on.

Prepare to Get Moving

Just as you did with planning, shopping for, and eating meals so that you'll have a heart-healthy food environment and healthy food choices right in your home, you need to think about and plan your future as a physically active person.

Exercise Clothes

Now it's time to search the clothes closets for exercise clothes. You do not need to make a trip to the store to buy something special. If you haven't been physically active, you'll begin by walking, so you'll need a pair of leggings, sweatpants, or shorts (if it's summer or you live in a warm climate), a T-shirt or tank top, sneakers or walking shoes with good support, and socks. Obviously, if you are exercising outside in cooler weather you will want to dress appropriately. You'll also need a bra that supports you well. Go through your closets and drawers to find what you'll need. It doesn't matter what you wear as long as it fits, is comfortable, and doesn't bind or chafe. If you don't find anything that fits, then go out and get yourself a new outfit (but don't spend $200 on a designer workout suit). You can also hit the local thrift store or check out the closets of others in your family. You probably have T-shirts galore, but if you need some shorts or sweats, get something inexpensive that's comfortable. You don't have to spend a fortune. Don't skimp on the shoes, however; they must have good support and allow you to walk comfortably. If your feet or legs hurt, you'll give up and won't gain the benefit of a walking program.

Exercise Equipment

There is no need to invest in any expensive equipment. If you have a pair of handheld dumbbells (two to five pounds), that's fine. Dust them off and put them in your bedroom, hallway, living room, or someplace in plain sight. If you can see them, you'll use them.

If you don't have dumbbells, there are plenty of household objects that will work instead. For example, take two empty one-liter soda bottles and fill them with water or sand. Better yet, use plastic half-gallon milk bottles; they come with a convenient handle, which makes them easier to grip. If the weights are too heavy, empty out some of the sand or water and add more as you gain strength.

Don't forget the cans in your cupboards. Cans of soup or vegetables can be pressed into double duty as weights, until they are needed for dinner.

If you decide you want dumbbells, they are very inexpensive and downright cheap if you go to one of the many stores that now sell used sports equipment. Mary got hers for 25¢ a pound. Thrift stores are also a good place to look, and if you live in the suburbs, garage sales can be a great source. Used exercise equipment is usually inexpensive and in great condition because the previous owner used it only once or twice.

Finally, designate a time and place in your home where you will exercise. Choose a time that will work best for you. In the morning when you get out of bed? While you watch television? Think about it and make sure you have the room to lift your weights and keep your "exercise tools" together in your selected area. If you have to go searching around for them each day, you will find something else to do instead. Don't set yourself up to fail.

There are many videos and books that can show you the exercises to do with your weights. We recommend *Mayo Clinic Fitness for Everybody*. This book has 150 easy-to-follow illustrated exercises. Consult their Web site to get started: www.bookstore.mayoclinic.com.

Facing Your Stress

Now that you've taken the first steps toward changing your diet and getting ready to be more active, it's time to turn your attention to decreasing the tension and stress in your life. Trust us, we don't want you to feel even more anxious or depressed when you think about how stressed you are, but living with high levels of stress is not good for your heart.

Helpful Facts About Stress

Stress is part of everyone's life and it is impossible to eliminate it totally. There is good stress and there is bad stress, and you need to learn to cope with both types because neither is good for your heart health.

You may be thinking, If stress is so bad for me, how can there be "good" stress? If nothing in your life causes you any stress or excitement, you may become bored or not feel challenged. You may never try anything new.

Some "good" stress—what you feel before an important job presentation or a test—may give you the extra energy you need to perform at your best. Good stress can be due to positive life-changing events like getting married or having a baby. But "bad" stress tends to be a constant worry over your job, school, or the health of a family member. It may cause you to have no energy and make it difficult for you to perform well.

If you are suffering from extreme, long-term, or chronic stress, your body will eventually wear itself down. If everything in your life causes you stress, you may need to discuss this with your doctor so you can make changes and improve your life. Just knowing what makes you stressed and how to better manage your stress can greatly improve your life.

Controlling or Changing Your Reaction to Stressors

Although you cannot eliminate either type of stress from your life, you can learn some very healthy ways to control the stress triggers, and you can change the way you react to the stress. Stress-reduction methods vary from simply taking time to cool out and listen to music, read a book, or enjoy a hobby to learning meditation, guided imagery, yoga, tai chi, or Pilates, or going for a walk. Sometimes sharing your feelings with a good friend or relative also works. Doing anything that takes your mind off what is bothering you works and will relieve stress.

If you find that nothing is able to relax you or make you feel less stressed, or that you commonly feel down or blue (especially if you're recovering from a heart attack or stroke), don't worry about it unless it goes on for too long and stops you from living a happy life. If you are at the point where the glass constantly looks half empty instead of half full, it's time to talk to your doctor, friends, family, or clergy, or consult a therapist, because you may be depressed.

Depression is a serious illness but it can be treated by a medical professional. You cannot treat depression yourself. Don't confuse depression with being overly stressed. Talk to someone (like your doctor) and get an honest assessment so that you can get the right kind of help.

Keep Track of Your Progress

You are going to have to keep track of your great progress, so we want you to go out and buy a notebook. You can treat yourself to a beautiful hand-bound journal or get a spiral notebook at the dollar store, whatever makes you happy. You are going to use this notebook as a journal for the next twenty-one days (weeks two, three, and four of the program—exercise, diet, and stress).

On page 1 of your notebook, list your personal risk factors (see Chapter 2). After each risk factor, make a positive statement, something that says how you intend to make a healthy change to eliminate or lower this particular risk. For example, if you don't get enough exercise, state something like, "I plan to walk for at least 15 minutes every day during my lunch hour." Once you're finished with each risk factor, sign that page. This is vital! Your signature will seal your commitment in writing. Your journal is meant to serve as a strong foundation to support you as you live up to your commitment to yourself every day. In fact, after you make your daily entry, read it out loud and then date and sign the page as proof that you heard it. You may want to do this with a friend. After she signs her page, then you can sign her page too, and vice versa. You can help each other and make a great team! Having a buddy to go through this process can be very powerful and effective.

Schedule an Appointment with Your Doctor or Nurse-Practitioner

Take your list of your personal risk factors with you when you see your doctor or nurse-practitioner. By knowing your specific risk factors, you can work with your medical professional to understand exactly where you stand in terms of your health. Maybe your blood pressure is not that high, but you still need to pay attention to it and try and lower it, maybe you need to be taking a medication, or maybe you're more overweight than you thought. Knowing your personal health status will empower you to start taking positive small steps to eliminate your chances of ever having a heart attack.

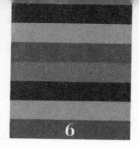

Week Two: Step 1:
Get Moving!

*P*utting on extra weight is so easy. An extra five pounds a year is not so difficult to gain, especially once we pass the age of thirty-five when, for most of us, our metabolism slows down. So if you weigh 130 pounds at age thirty-five and pack on five pounds a year, by age forty you'll weigh 155 and by age fifty you'll weigh 205! Of course that's an extreme, but it's still possible and we've seen women who have done just that.

This chapter will show you how easy it is to put on weight and how easy it can be to take it off, once you put your mind to it. Of course you will change your usual routine by adding exercise, but trust us, once you start to move around, the pounds will come off and you'll feel and look much better—and you'll be motivated to continue the program.

Why We're So Fat

It is estimated that we eat only a couple hundred calories more a day than we did thirty years ago. If this is true, then why is America now the land of obesity? The problem lies in the fact that people are not as active as they were thirty years ago. Granted, today we have junk food, fast food, packaged food, and many other forms of concentrated calorie food to eat, but we wouldn't be so overweight as a nation if we just moved around more and burned off some of those calories.

For most Americans, a typical day consists of running errands from their car. We've got drive-through banks, pharmacies, fast-food restaurants, coffee shops, doughnut shops, florists, and even dry cleaners. In some states, you don't have to get out to pump your own gas, and even if you do, you can check out at the pump, so you don't need to walk to the cashier anymore. At home we've got riding mowers and self-propelled vacuum cleaners. For those of us who live in the city, we don't have to expend energy cooking or doing dishes. We can just dial the phone and have any type of food we feel like eating delivered to our door. Not only that, in America, we have an unlimited choice of food and can have anything we want anytime we want—and we often do. We are also a nation of sedentary people. Even at the office we eat at our desks or take the elevator to the cafeteria.

We've paid a high price for being lazy. Along with obesity come all the usual illnesses—diabetes, high blood pressure, and high cholesterol—that contribute to coronary heart disease, which often leads to heart attack or stroke. We can change this by just getting up and moving around—it doesn't take much. Before you learn how to make changes, let us give you some facts that you might find hard to believe.

One recent study published in the *Journal of the American Medical Association* found that obese adults who lost just 7 percent of their weight (that amounts to 16 pounds for a 220-pound woman) by doing moderate-intensity physical exercise for six months (this means exercising just two or three times a week) shaved 500 calories a day from their diet and improved their major blood vessel function by about 80 percent. These women all showed improvement in blood sugar and cholesterol levels. They gained all of these benefits just from doing moderate exercise, something we can all do.

Not Exercising Is Our Biggest Mistake!

Exercise doesn't have to be all or nothing. Overestimating how much exercise is needed is the primary reason why many women don't exercise at all. Many women we've spoken to incorrectly assume that since they don't have an hour a day every day to devote to serious athletic training, there is no point doing any exercise. This is the worst mistake any of us can make, because it is so far from the truth. Every little bit helps. And when it comes to getting moving, doing *something* is always better than doing nothing.

We frequently mention that taking small steps does make a difference, and exercise is the perfect model for that promise. Taking small steps as you add an activity like walking to your daily routine can literally get you on the road to a heart-healthy future.

Any physical exercise or activity has a number of benefits that directly affect your heart.

- It makes your heart stronger. A stronger heart can pump blood more efficiently.
- It lowers blood pressure. When the heart works more efficiently, it has to work less, which means less pressure is placed on your arteries.
- It increases and improves the condition of your veins and arteries (circulatory system).
- It may even decrease the body's release of a hormone that raises blood pressure, because exercise helps to constrict arteries by increasing the heart rate.
- It helps to improve your mood. You are feeling better within the first few days because you are active. Try it and see (and feel) what we mean!

Ten Minutes a Day

A recent study published in the *Journal of the American Medical Association* showed that when overweight or obese women who previously were inactive exercised an average of one hour and twelve minutes per week, they improved their fitness and heart health. Ten minutes a day is all you need to *begin* to get the benefits of exercise. The choice is yours. We say, "Go for it!" Deciding to exercise is the single best thing you can do for your heart (besides quitting smoking) because its benefits affect so many areas of your well-being.

If you think you don't have the time to exercise, consider how many minutes you fritter away sitting and not moving as you

- do your nails
- leaf through a magazine
- stop off for a latte or café con leche on the way to or from work
- watch TV
- read or do crosswords or sudoku
- talk on the phone
- sit at the computer

We could go on, but you get the picture. The trick is to move around instead of sitting. If you set your mind to adding exercise to your life, you'll find time to do it, even if you have to schedule it in your daily calendar—it's just as valid as your other appointments—or take time from your lunch hour, or schedule ten minutes for an after-dinner walk with your spouse, child, friend, or neighbor.

The Benefits of Walking Are Free

Consider this: An eight-year study of more than seventy thousand women found that brisk walking and vigorous exercise were associated with substantial reductions in the incidence of heart attacks in women. Even light to moderate activity was associated with lower rates of heart disease. At least one hour of walking per week reduced the risk of heart disease. Women who walked thirty minutes a day had significantly lower risk of premature death than those who rarely exercised. You don't need an expensive gym or fancy clothes; you just need a pair of good shoes and a few minutes a day.

Get Moving—Ten Minutes at a Time

Your plan this week is to spend at least ten minutes each day walking or doing some other type of active movement. If you can't take time during the day, get up ten minutes earlier or take some time after dinner. Here are some suggestions—we're sure you can think of more.

- Park your car farther away from the store or the office. If you take the bus or subway, walk to a stop farther away from your home or work.
- Don't use the drive-through window. Park your car and walk into the store.
- Go for a walk at lunch.
- Get up earlier and walk before work.

- Make walking a family affair. Walk to the park or around the block after dinner.
- Walk your dog or volunteer to walk a neighbor's dog.
- Garden, rake, mow the lawn, cut the hedges.
- Take a long route to your destination (even if it's in a shopping mall).

If you live or work in an area that isn't safe to walk in, then you must be creative about how you can add exercise to your day.

- Exercise while you watch TV.
- Pace the room while you're on the phone.
- Take the stairs when you can. Even if you work on the twentieth floor, you can get off the elevator on nineteen and walk up one flight. As your comfort level increases, get off at eighteen or seventeen.
- Use the bathroom one floor up or one floor down at work and take the stairs to get there.
- Walk up the escalator; don't just stand there.
- Join in the early morning walk at your neighborhood shopping mall (call the mall to see what time the walkers meet).
- Take your family and walk around the mall (leave the credit cards at home).

Walking Healthy

As with starting any exercise program, be sure to check with your doctor before you begin walking. If you've been

leading a sedentary lifestyle, ten minutes a day could prove
to be a real workout until you do it for a while. Once ten
minutes is comfortable, add a few more minutes so that
you are challenged but not exhausted by your walk.

If you think that there's nothing to know about walking, think again. In order to get the full health benefit, there
are a couple of things to keep in mind. When you're walking for exercise, pay attention to *how* you're walking.

- **Let your heel hit the ground first,** rolling onto the ball of
  your foot and ending with a strong push off the toes.
- **Walk quickly** if you can, rather than taking longer strides.
- **Maintain good posture.** Look straight ahead with your chin
  level (not pointed up high or tucked into your chest). Keep your
  shoulders and upper back relaxed, but don't slouch. Stand up
  straight and keep that rump in. Aim for a slight natural arch in
  your back.
- **Pull in your abdominal muscles gently** as you walk to
  strengthen your abs. This technique also reduces lower-back pain.
- **Swing your arms naturally at your sides** (this burns an
  extra five to ten calories). Follow an imaginary line in the center
  of the pavement in front of you. You can really get moving: Bend
  your arms at the elbows and swing them from your waist to
  your chest in step with your foot movements. Your hands should
  reach just below your chin and your forearms should brush your
  hips. Remember those dumbbells? Take them on your walk and
  give your arms a workout too.

- **Breathe deeply.** If you find yourself getting short of breath, slow down and walk only on flat surfaces.
- **Walk to the music.** Take along your MP3 or CD player or radio. If you don't have one, borrow one from your kids. Plug in those headphones (but keep the volume down and watch out for traffic you might not be able to hear). Keep pace with the beat.
- **Walk with a purpose**, as if you have an important destination in mind—don't meander. You want to raise your heartbeat and feel that you've done some exercise.
- **Take your pulse.** Two easy places to find your pulse are at the inside of your wrist on either hand along the thumb side. Immediately after exercise, place the first two fingers of one hand (not your thumb) on an artery and count the number of beats in ten seconds. Multiply that number by 6 to determine your heart rate in beats per minute. (See below for determining your ideal heart rate.)

Monitor Your Heart Rate

You may feel as if you're getting lots of exercise as you huff and puff up and down the stairs at work or walk with the mall walkers. But in order to know if you are you working your heart too hard or not hard enough, you need to know how to monitor your heart rate. You can't tell how hard your heart is working by how much you sweat; some women get drenched when they work out while others are barely damp.

When you exercise, your heart beats faster as your muscles require more blood and oxygen, and the harder the exercise, the faster your heart beats. That's why monitoring is a great way to figure out how intense your workout actually is.

To determine a safe "target heart rate zone"—the number of beats per minute that your heart should beat during aerobic exercise—you must do a little math.

First, figure out your "maximum heart rate." This is the absolute highest rate for someone your age while exercising. But unless you are ready for the Olympics, your rate should never get this high. This is related to your age, because as you get older, your heart slows down slightly. To find your maximum heart rate, subtract your age from 220.

Second, you need to find out your "target heart rate zone." For most healthy individuals, the target range is 50 to 80 percent of your maximum heart rate. To find the low end of your target heart rate range (50 percent), multiply .5 × your maximum heart rate (220 minus your age in years). To find the high end of the range (80 percent), multiply .8 × your maximum heart rate.

Here's what the calculation would look like for a fifty-year-old woman:

Maximum heart rate:

$$220 - 50 = 170$$

50% target heart rate (low):

$$170 \times .5 = 85$$

80% target heart rate (high):

$$170 \times .8 = 136$$

In other words, a fifty-year-old woman would have a target heart rate zone of 85 to 136 beats per minute.

Knowing your range can help you determine how hard you should be exercising or if you're overdoing it or slacking. When you're starting out, aim for the low end of the zone and add more intense workouts as the weeks pass. If you're more fit, aim for the higher end of the zone.

Of course, this assumes that your heart is healthy. If you have heart disease or you're taking medication that affects your heart rate, consult your doctor for guidance on how much and what type of exercise is best for you.

Hydrate

Because walking is a workout, be sure you hydrate your body. Drink an eight-ounce glass of water about ten minutes before your walk and then drink another glass or two when you get home. If you are walking in heat, dress in lightweight and light-colored clothing, wear sunscreen and sunglasses, and carry water with you. You also can get dehydrated when it's cold, so don't forget water when temperatures are cooler.

Safety Concerns

Never leave home without a whistle, a cell phone, and a flashlight (if you are walking after dark). Always tell someone where and when you'll be walking and when you expect to be back. Better yet, enlist a walking buddy. It's safer and more enjoyable to walk together. Also, if you've made a commitment to walk with someone else, you are less likely to skip your walk.

If you're walking in an urban area, you'll be able to walk on the sidewalks. But for those of you who live in the country or the suburbs, always walk *facing* oncoming traffic. That way you'll be able to see anything coming toward you (and have time get out of the way if necessary). Don't walk after dark in an area you aren't familiar with, and walk in a safe place. Wear bright-colored clothing and white or reflective bands so drivers can see you.

Reward Yourself

After your first week, treat yourself to something that will enhance your exercise regime. Rent an exercise CD or tape or borrow one from of the library (for free), or buy a fitness magazine or a healthy treat. As you progress, you can reward yourself with a spiffy new pair of shoes, exercise clothes, or a fancy water bottle. Enlist your family too. When they ask what you would like for your birthday or Mother's Day, ask for a subscription to a walking magazine or healthy eating magazine—the gift and benefits will last all year.

When You'll See Results

You won't have to wait long to see the benefits of exercise. By the end of the first week you should notice some changes, like having more energy, sleeping better, and a clearer mind. Your appetite may also be easier to control. Don't expect to lose much weight right away, but if you continue walking you will lose weight gradually, which should be a reward in itself. Slow weight loss stays off longer than rapid weight loss. Weight gain usually occurs slowly over time, so don't expect it to come off quicker than it was put on. Keep up the good work and keep moving!

Log Your Progress

You may prefer to keep track of the number of steps you walk each day and use that as a measuring stick. If you want to count steps, you will need to buy a pedometer. Put it on first thing in the morning and count your steps throughout the day. Aim for three thousand steps a day, and increase gradually to get to ten thousand per day at least four days a week.

In your journal, keep track of your progress. You can add a section to your journal that charts your exercise, and check off each day you succeed. Also include a section where you can discuss your mood and how you were feeling physically before and after you exercised. This will help you discover a pattern as you look back over the next few weeks. Before you started exercising, you might have been feeling happy but tired after being out late last night. After you started exercise, you'll note that you feel happy and energetic! Keeping these records can really help you see how you're coming along and encourage you to keep at it.

You may prefer to download a walking journal off the Internet. Search "free walking log" or "free walking journal" and you will be directed to many sites. Pick the log or journal format you prefer. Enlist the help of your kids or friends if you are not a computer whiz—maybe they will keep a log too. This can create some positive family competition.

You will continue to walk your minimum of ten minutes each day while you learn about heart-healthy eating in week three of the program.

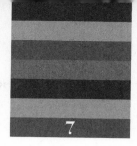

Week Three: Step 2: Simple Steps to Healthier Eating

$\mathcal{T}$his chapter is not about dieting or denying yourself familiar, comforting food. Instead it will show you how to eat in moderation and give suggestions on how to prepare traditional foods in a healthy way.

We need to eat to live, but when we eat too much of the wrong types of food, that works against us and actually shortens our life. We're sure that you already know this, but the mystery remains: If so many people are aware that being overweight or eating unhealthy food can raise blood pressure, aggravate diabetes, clog arteries, and make us fat, why don't we all just change our diet to a healthier one? It's just not that easy because of the complicated relationship we have with food.

In many cultures, food is used as a way to bring families together, express love and show that we care, and let others know that we are doing well in life. In some cultures, being overweight is actually proof that life is good.

African-American and Latino cuisines, although they taste great, have not contributed in a positive way to the health of their members. It's not that other cultures don't also consider food important. The Italians and French, for example, make eating the center of family and social life. But one important difference is that, for many years, these two cuisines have been making light versions of traditional favorites. Italian food isn't always pasta with a heavy sauce. Now it is often whole wheat pasta topped with fresh tomato and vegetable sauce. Even the cheeses are now made with skim or part-skim milk. The French led the way toward cooking light. At first it was a joke because the portions were minuscule, but that has changed as the French have discovered ways to substitute ingredients lower in fat and carbohydrates. African Americans and Latinos have been slow to jump on this healthy bandwagon.

African-American Cuisine

African-American cuisine was, for the most part, invented in America. When African Americans first came to the United States, food was limited, and because Blacks were unable to find traditional ingredients, they used what they had at hand. They made tasty dishes that used a lot of healthy ingredients like corn, potatoes (white and sweet), collards, spinach, and root vegetables, along with what meat was available, usually chicken and cheaper cuts of meat, like spareribs and neck bones. Over time, African-American food developed diverse flavors as the cuisine included not only traditional flavors from Africa but also flavors from the West Indies and North America. In the mid-1960s, African Americans were more than twice as likely as Caucasians to eat a diet that met the American Heart Association's recommended daily guidelines for fruit, vegetables, fat, and fiber. However, by the mid-1990s, the diet of African Americans had changed and now consisted of more fried and processed foods with fewer portions of fruits and vegetables.

While African-American cuisine includes many nutritious and heart-healthy items such as beans (rich in protein and low in fat), green and yellow leafy vegetables, (filled with vitamins and antioxidants), and fish and poultry, many of the common cooking methods—deep frying; seasoning with bacon, ham, or ham hocks; adding gravy; adding salt—negate the heart-healthy benefits and add fat and calories. Heart-healthy foods such as red beans, yams, cornmeal, rice, fish, chicken, Black-eyed peas, and collard greens have excellent nutritional values when prepared with low-fat methods and seasoned with natural spices instead of salt.

This heritage of rich food has helped to put African Americans at the top of the list for heart disease, high blood pressure, diabetes, and stroke. These heart disease risk factors are all affected by diet. Leading the list is hypertension and its relation to salt. Hypertension is very common in African-American women, and about 75 percent of African Americans with hypertension are salt sensitive, which means that their blood pressure is likely to increase with increasing salt intake. Therefore, reducing salt intake is of great importance in controlling blood pressure in African-American women. Today, African Americans make up a large part of our fast-food nation. Unhealthy diet plus inactivity (as we saw in Chapter 6) is a lethal combination.

Simple Tips for Heart-Healthy African-American Cuisine

It is okay to have traditionally cooked African-American foods once in a while. However, many of the traditional dishes can be made with less fat, less salt, and fewer calories and still maintain the traditional flavor.

- Reduce the fat. Grill, sauté, and steam and avoid frying.
- Remove the skin, and you can still enjoy baked fish and chicken.
- Substitute turkey bacon, ham, or Canadian bacon for regular bacon.
- Switch from cooking with butter, margarine, and lard to a healthy oil like canola, olive, or safflower.
- Cook beans with lean ham or chicken parts instead of ham hocks or other pork products.

- Steam greens and other vegetables and add onions and peppers. Add a drop of liquid smoke to provide flavor. Add okra to stews and soups to thicken them, instead of cream or butter.
- Use salt substitutes (Salt Sense, Papa Dash, Mrs. Dash) in place of salt. Use onion, garlic, or salt-free seasoning blends for seasoning. Add Black or red pepper, onion, and garlic as seasonings instead of salt.

Latin Cuisine

The Latino culture also has food at its center. Family gatherings, religious holidays, baptisms, communions, and weddings are all times to get together and cook lavish feasts.

The traditional Latin diet has much in common with the heart-healthy Mediterranean diet. Although Latin America spans eighteen nations, the traditional Latin diet includes fruits, vegetables, legumes, beans, nuts, whole grains, and tubers (potatoes are one type of tuber). Legumes, beans, and nuts are important to heart health as they are high in fiber (great for helping to lower cholesterol and helping to manage blood sugar levels in those with diabetes) and are good sources of protein. The Latin diet also includes fish, shellfish, poultry, dairy, and plant oils (olive oil and soy). The traditional Latin family consumed red meat, eggs, and sweets only about once a week.

Unfortunately, in today's world, very few Latin Americans follow traditional eating habits and have adopted the

American-influenced diet, which is high in added fats, fatty foods, huge portions, and rich desserts. This has led to an increase in the number of Latinos with diet-related health problems. In fact, more Latinos are obese than any other culture, with Mexicans leading the way.

Therefore, going back to the basic traditional Latin American style of cooking and eating can lead to a decrease in the number of women at risk for heart disease. Making heart-smart substitutions at home and at restaurants can have a powerful impact on the fight against heart disease.

Simple Heart-Healthy Latin Cooking Tips

- Increase the amount of vegetables and decrease the amount of meat in a recipe.
- Bake, broil, or grill all food instead of frying. Limit red meat to once a week and instead cook chicken, lean pork, fish, and seafood.
- Serve fresh fruit instead of fruit nectars.
- Use low-fat cheese in recipes and eat low-fat cream cheese.
- Cut back on the sugar or use sugar substitutes.
- Cook with skim or 1% milk instead of whole milk.
- Choose corn or whole wheat tortillas instead of those made with white flour.
- Replace lard with canola or safflower oil.
- Use the low-fat or skim varieties of condensed or evaporated milk.
- Substitute quesadillas; choose grilled marinated chicken fajitas; a one-cup serving of cooked beans, peas, or lentils has the propor-

tionate amount of protein as a 3-ounce serving of meat, poultry, or fish.

Recently, the "nuevo Latino" cuisine has become popular in the United States. A new generation of Latino chefs from all over Latin America are creating new, exciting, and healthier combinations using some of the ancient traditions of Latin cuisine.

Heart-healthy choices such as fresh fish seviche, yucca fries, Mexican corn soup, *ropa vieja* (meat stew), and Black beans and rice are included in the nuevo Latino cusine. For more information, go to www.foodnetwork.com and take a look at the cookbook *Latin Lover Lite* by Chef LaLa, which has many heart-smart recipes.

The High Price of Living on a Budget

It is well established that diet plays an important role in heart disease, the leading cause of death in the United States. Diets high in fat and cholesterol raise the amount of fat and cholesterol in the blood and increase risk of developing heart disease. Several studies have reported that Americans with low incomes have the greatest risk for heart disease, which is another reason why people of color (and women of color, in particular) have such a high rate of health problems.

Today's lower-income women tend to be Black or Latina. They have the great skill of being creative when preparing food on a limited budget. Unfortunately, less

expensive foods also tend to be high in fat and carbohydrates. Fast food falls right into this category of inexpensive and fattening. There is quite a variety of fast-food
choices for as little as one dollar, although they aren't necessarily healthy.

Healthy Traditions: Ways to Make Favorite Foods Healthy

You don't need to give up all of your favorite foods, but
you will have to modify the recipes and the way you cook
them, and you may not be able to eat some dishes as often
as you'd like. Trust us when we say that this is a change
you can live with that will allow you to live a long healthy
life. You'll also be able to teach your children and grand-
children new ways to make old favorites and start a new
tradition.

Kesha and Calvin lived with their two children and
with Kesha's mother, Hildreth. Hildreth did all the shopping and cooking—barbecued ribs, fried chicken, fried
pork, collard greens, and buttery corn bread. That all
changed when a free health screening revealed that Kesha
had dangerously high blood pressure and cholesterol. The
information we gave her about high blood pressure, obesity, and stroke was scary. The family started on our five-
week, three-step program, making just a few small changes
at a time. First, they ate fried food only three times a week
instead of five or six. Hildreth started cutting down on salt

and replaced corn oil with safflower oil. When collard greens were on the menu, she omitted the pork and lard. Next, they served fruit three nights a week, instead of peach cobbler or ice cream sundaes. After five weeks, Kesha's blood pressure and cholesterol were still a bit high but no longer dangerous.

Your Heart-Smart Eating Plan

In week one you restocked the pantry, fridge, and freezer with healthy foods and snacks. Now we're going to show you how to incorporate them into a heart-smart eating plan. At the risk of sounding like a broken record, we want to reassure you that this is not a rigid or restrictive diet. We want you to enjoy your new way of cooking and eating, because if you like it, you'll continue on it for the rest of what should be a long and healthy life full of good things to cook and eat.

The following steps outline a heart-smart eating plan that is based on moderation. The bottom line: If you take in fewer calories than you burn off, you will lose weight and become healthier in the long run. You'll get most of your calories from fruits and vegetables, but you'll still be able to eat meat and fish and use oil for cooking and flavoring. Doing things a little differently in the kitchen can add excitement and newfound pleasure to cooking. You'll be cutting way back on the sugar, though, but it won't be banished from your life.

The Five Basic Steps for Healthy Eating at Every Meal

1. Pay Attention to Portion Control and Don't Help Yourself to Seconds

Your watchwords are *moderation* and *balance*. Paying attention to the size of your portions will help you decrease calories. Portions have gotten larger at most restaurants, including fast-food restaurants. The problem for most of us is that these big portions now look normal.

In order to help you eyeball and visualize the size of the portions you should be eating without carrying around a scale or calorie counter, use your hand.

- 1 closed fist (or a tennis ball or baseball) = 1 cup of vegetables, pasta, rice, cereal, or cut-up fruit
- 1 open palm, minus the fingers (or 1 deck of cards) = 2–3 ounces of meat, fish, chicken
- 1 thumb = 1 ounce of cheese
- 1 thumb tip = 1 teaspoon of margarine or peanut/almond butter
- 3 thumb tips = 1 tablespoon / 12 grams
- 1 dime = 1 gram
- 1 die = 1 teaspoon / 4 grams

Judging serving sizes is a skill that you'll learn quickly. If you are served a larger portion at a restaurant, take half of your entrée home in a doggie bag and save it for another meal.

2. Increase Your Daily Intake of Fresh Fruits and Vegetables and Foods High in Soluble Fiber

All fruits, vegetables, grains, and legumes tend to be low in fat and low in cholesterol. In addition, most are excellent sources of dietary fiber, complex carbohydrates, and vitamins.

Remember, though, it depends on how they are prepared. If you take healthy vegetables or bananas and deep-fry them, they are no longer a healthy choice. Overall, most Americans eat only 15 grams of fiber a day, when the recommended average is 20–35 grams of fiber daily for adults.

GET READY TO "ROUGH IT!"

Fiber is often referred to as bulk or roughage. Fiber is good for your digestive tract and it can also help lower cholesterol.

The general term *fiber* usually refers to carbohydrates that cannot be digested. Fiber can absorb many times its weight in water, resulting in softer, bulkier stools. You need to drink enough fluids, as fiber absorbs more water than other foods. A diet high in fiber helps keep food moving through the intestine by expanding the inside walls of the colon, which eases the passage of waste. The added bulk helps you feel full with much less food. Fibrous foods often take longer to chew and can help slow down the pace of eating your meal.

Fiber can be broken down into two categories. Soluble

fiber is partially broken down in water. When soluble fiber is a regular part of your daily diet, it can actually help lower cholesterol. Some common foods that contain soluble fiber are oatmeal; oat bran; barley; nuts; seeds; legumes such as dried peas, chickpeas, kidney beans, Black beans, pinto beans, lentils; apples; pears; strawberries; and blueberries.

Insoluble fiber cannot be broken down in water. It does not seem to have the same lowering effect on cholesterol, but it is still an important part of your diet as it helps promote normal bowel function. The best sources of insoluble fiber are whole grains such as whole wheat bread, couscous, brown rice, and bulgur. Whole grains haven't had their bran and germ removed by milling, which makes them a great source of fiber and nutrients.

However, it can be tricky to find a whole grain food. Food companies often make it appear that a product contains whole grains when it doesn't. Look for items listed on the label with the main ingredient whole wheat, whole oats, whole rye, or some other whole-grain cereal. If the label simply says made with wheat flour, it may not be the whole grain.

Vegetables also contain insoluble fiber. Include carrots, zucchini, celery, tomatoes, broccoli, pumpkin, squash, cucumbers, cabbage, brussels sprouts, turnips, and cauliflower in your diet. (Note that canned vegetables often contain a lot of salt, which you may want to limit, especially if you have high blood pressure. Buy the no-salt-added versions and rinse them in water before heating.)

3. Eat Fish at Least Twice a Week and Cut down on Red Meat

Fish is a great alternative to high-fat meats as a source of protein. Cod, tuna, and halibut are lower in fat and cholesterol than many meat and poultry choices.

Omega-3 polyunsaturated fatty acids help reduce the risk of death from coronary artery disease by decreasing cardiac arrhythmia, lowering levels of triglycerides (fats) in your blood, slowing the growth of plaque in the arteries, and slightly lowering blood pressure. Omega-3s are found in fish, especially salmon, mackerel, sardines, trout, bluefish, albacore tuna, and herring. The American Heart Association recommends that you eat at least two 3-ounce servings of this type of fish a week to reap these benefits.

Grill, bake, or poach the fish (frying destroys the health benefits) and don't add creamy sauces. Just cook with little olive oil and season with lemon and garlic for a simple and delicious, healthy meal.

4. Reduce and Limit Salt, Unhealthy Fat, and Sugar

SALT

Consuming excess salt is one of the main causes of high blood pressure and other related heart diseases. A study published in the *British Medical Journal* in April 2007 demonstrated that reducing the level of salt in the diet leads to a reduced risk of heart attacks and stroke. Over 80 percent of salt intake is from processed foods, which contain what are often called "hidden salts." Therefore, it is important to check all food labels for salt content. The American Heart Association encourages women to become salt detectives and seek low-salt foods, ones that have 140 milligrams or less sodium per serving.

Tips for Cutting Salt

- Choose frozen and canned foods, soups, cereals, baked goods, and other processed foods labeled "reduced-sodium," "sodium-free," "no salt added," or "unsalted."
- Check food labels for total sodium content 140 mg or less per serving. Note that sodium may also be listed as monosodium glutamate (MSG). Limit consumption of high-sodium condiments and foods such as soy sauce, steak sauce, Worcestershire sauce, flavored seasoning salts, pickles, olives, anchovies, cured meats, bacon, hot dogs, sausage, bologna, ham, salami, nuts, sauerkraut, tomato and other vegetable juices, and cheese.
- Don't cook with salt or add salt to the food on your plate. Instead use pepper, garlic, lemon, or other spices for flavor. Replace salt with herbs and spices or some of the salt-free seasonings like Mrs. Dash, but be careful of other packaged spice blends that often contain salt or salt products.
- Rinse canned meats, vegetables, and capers in plain water to remove some of the sodium.

- When eating out, order steamed, grilled, baked, boiled, and broiled foods and request no salt, sauce, or cheese be added.

SATURATED FAT

Saturated fat is the one true dietary demon that we should make a conscious effort to cut back on. Saturated fat is the most potent type of cholesterol-raising fat in our diet. You should eat no more than 20 grams of saturated fat a day, according to the U.S. Department of Agriculture's 2007 Dietary Guidelines.

Tips for Cutting Saturated Fat

- Choose lean cuts of beef and pork (look for "loin" or "round" on the package in the grocery store).
- Trim as much visible fat as possible from meat and remove the skin from poultry before cooking.
- Skim the fat from the top of soups. To make this easier, if time allows, place the soup in the refrigerator. After it cools, you can easily scrape the solidified fat off the top. Instead of meat, make soups with protein-rich foods such as kidney beans, Black beans, pinto beans, lentils, and chickpeas.
- Make healthy refried beans by mashing them with low-sodium chicken broth or some of the cooking water and refrying in a small amount of canola oil or no-stick spray rather than lard.
- Avoid deep-frying and instead sauté vegetables in low-salt chicken or beef broth or diced fresh tomatoes.

- Replace fats such as bacon grease and butter with olive or canola oil.
- Steam vegetables, adding a few spices for flavor.
- Use oil and vinegar rather than bottled dressings on salads because this is lower in fat and calories.
- Replace heavy cream sauces and butter with low-fat or nonfat sour cream and serve sauces on the side. Don't add butter or margarine to food—you may be surprised at how good fresh sweet corn is without it.
- Eat your vegetables raw with some low-calorie salad dressing or salsa.

Trans Fats

Trans fats are monounsaturated or polyunsaturated fats that have been altered by partial hydrogenation to make them solid at room temperature. Trans fats make food products last longer. The Food and Drug Administration (FDA) requires that all packaged food list the trans fat content. Look for the words "partially hydrogenated oil" or "vegetable shortening" on the ingredients list.

Some common sources of trans fatty acid are baked goods such as doughnuts and pastry, deep-fried foods such as fried chicken and french fries, and imitation cheese. Snack chips, cookies, and crackers often contain high amounts of trans fat.

Trans-fatty acids are formed when a liquid fat is converted to solid fat. The resulting hydrogenated fats can increase levels of LDL. They can also decrease levels of HDL.

Finally, trans fat can make blood platelets stickier, which in turn can accelerate the progression of atherosclerosis and increase the risk for cardiovascular events such as a heart attack and stroke.

Foods with less than 0.5 gram of trans fat per serving can claim to be trans fat free on the label. This is misleading because if you eat more than one serving of some of these "trans fat free" foods, you will actually be eating a significant amount of trans fat that can easily add up. So don't believe what a label says on the front—check the ingredients, and if it says "partially hydrogenated oil," don't buy it.

Because there is no safe limit for trans fats, you should eat as little of them as possible. The American Heart Association recommends limiting the combined amount of trans and saturated fats to less than 10 percent of total calories consumed daily. Snack foods are the main source of trans fat in your diet.

Tips for Cutting Trans Fats

- Cut back on foods containing partially hydrogenated vegetable oils.
- Limit the amount of solid fats—butter, margarine, and shortening. Use liquid canola oil or olive oil in place of hard margarine, vegetable oil or shortening, and lard.
- Top your baked sweet potato with low-fat yogurt, low-fat cottage cheese, or salsa instead of butter or margarine.
- Use sugar-free fruit spread on your whole wheat toast or muffin instead of butter or margarine.

- Limit cakes, cookies, crackers, pastries, pies, muffins, doughnuts, and french fries made with partially hydrogenated or saturated fats.

SUGAR—EMPTY CALORIES!

One eight-ounce glass of soda contains eighteen tablespoons of sugar! You'll be amazed at how fast you can lose weight if you stop drinking sugary beverages. These drinks tend to be low in vitamins and minerals, and the calories add up quickly but do not make you feel full, which could tempt you into eating and drinking more than you need and you'll gain weight. Soda is particularly bad. Full-sugar soft drinks are also linked with drinking less milk and fruit juice, along with an increased risk of type 2 diabetes.

Carbonated soft drinks are the single largest source of calories in the American diet. Companies annually manufacture enough soda pop to provide more than fifty-two gallons to every man, woman, and child in the United States.

Sugars are listed on the nutrition labels in many ways. Look for sucrose, glucose, fructose, maltose, dextrose, corn syrups, high-fructose corn syrup, concentrated fruit juice, and honey. Read the ingredient list carefully and choose items that don't have added sugars in their first four listed ingredients.

5. Eat a Variety of Foods at Every Meal— Your Plate Should Be Colorful!

The American Heart Association recommends that you color your plate to prevent heart disease. A balanced heart-healthy diet includes foods from all the major food groups, with particular emphasis on vegetables, fruits, and whole grains. This translates into two cups of fruit and two and a half cups of vegetables per day for a typical one thousand eight hundred-calorie intake, with higher or lower amounts depending on your individual calorie needs.

Your heart-healthy diet should be colorful, containing all five vegetable subgroups: dark green—spinach, collards, turnip greens, lettuce, kale, broccoli; orange—carrots, sweet potatoes, pumpkin, winter squash; legumes—dry beans, chickpeas, tofu; starch (in moderation)—corn, peas, white potatoes; other—tomatoes, cabbage, celery, cucumbers, onions, peppers, green beans, cauliflower, mushrooms, summer squash.

In addition, aim for six whole-grain products per day.

HOW MUCH TO EAT

Since you now know what you can eat, we'll give you the guidelines on how much to eat.

Fruit and Vegetables: 5 servings per day

I serving =

    I piece of fruit (apple, banana, peach, etc.)

    ½ cup berries

    8 ounces (I cup) cup of leafy greens (raw or cooked)

    ½ cup of nonleafy vegetables (raw or cooked)

    6 ounces of fruit or vegetable juice

Protein: 2 servings per day

I serving =

    3 ounces of cooked lean meat (chicken without skin,
        turkey, lean beef) or fish

    4 ounces of cooked lentils or other beans

    I egg

    2 tablespoons peanut butter

Dairy: 3 servings per day

I serving =

    I cup of low-fat or fat-free milk

    I cup of low-free or fat-free yogurt

    4 ounces of low-fat cottage cheese

    2 ounces of cheese

Whole Grain: 6 servings per day

I serving =

    I slice whole grain bread

    I cup of breakfast cereal (compare boxes for those with
        less sugar)

4 ounces of cooked oatmeal

4 ounces of cooked whole wheat pasta

½ cup of cooked brown rice

½ whole wheat bagel

Eat Healthier Versions of the Foods You Love

We are fortunate to be living in the twenty-first century, especially when it comes to eating. Today we have sugar substitutes that taste good, and we have nonfat, low-fat, and reduced-fat milk, cheese, and ice cream. These advances make it so much easier to eat the foods we love but in healthier versions—just don't forget to keep the serving size in check!

Consider the following when you start your heart-healthy eating plan. In some cases, like substituting 1% or skim milk for whole milk in flan, for example, we doubt if your family will even notice.

- Replace processed cheese such as Colby, Cheez Whiz, Velveeta, and most packaged presliced or pimiento cheese with nonfat mild cheese, soy cheese, or 1% milk cheese.
- Replace whole-milk cheese with skim, 1%, or nonfat milk cheese or soy cheese.
- Replace regular full-fat ice cream with soy ice cream, low-fat or fat-free ice cream, or frozen yogurt.
- Replace regular cream cheese with nonfat or ½ fat cream cheese or with soy cream cheese.

- Replace regular mayonnaise with light or diet mayonnaise, or Vegenaise.
- Replace regular salad dressing with reduced-calorie, fat-free dressings or oil and vinegar.
- Replace white bread with whole wheat bread or whole-grain bread.
- Replace Cream of Wheat with oatmeal.
- Replace cornflakes with All-Bran or other whole-grain cereals.
- Replace white potatoes with yams or sweet potatoes.
- Replace whole eggs with egg whites or egg substitutes.
- Replace white rice with brown rice.
- Replace white sugar with sugar substitutes or at least cut down the amount of sugar you eat and cook with. Some sugar substitutes, like Splenda granular, can be used cup for cup like sugar, or you can substitute up to three-quarters of the sugar in a recipe with it.
- Replace all sugared sodas with diet sodas. Better yet, reach for plain or sparkling water or a flavored water.
- Replace white pasta with whole wheat pasta.
- Replace salted nuts with raw almonds or walnuts.
- Replace regular beef and pork with fish, skinless chicken, tofu, beans, or leaner cuts of beef.

Oils, Butter, Margarine

Margarine is made from vegetable oils, so it contains no cholesterol.

Margarine is also higher in "good" fats—polyunsaturated and monounsaturated—than butter is.

But not all margarines are created equal—some may even be worse than butter. Most margarine is hydrogenated, which adds unhealthy trans fats. A good rule of thumb is that the more solid the margarine, the more trans fats it contains. So stick margarines usually have more trans fats than do tub margarines.

Throw away the lard and the bacon fat and start using healthy oils for cooking. Canola, corn, safflower, soybean, and olive oil are all good choices. Use liquid vegetable oils that have no more than 2 grams of saturated fat per tablespoon when cooking.

There are also spreads—such as Benecol and Take Control—that contain phytosterols, a natural plant compound that has been shown to reduce LDL (bad) cholesterol levels by as much as 15 percent when eaten in recommended amounts. They are available in most local supermarkets.

Now that you have become heart smart regarding what you eat and how much to eat, you can add healthy eating to exercising a minimum of ten minutes each day. Step three of the heart-smart plan is to lessen your stress. Congratulations on the changes you have kept thus far. Remember to keep your mind on your goals and you will become healthy, strong, energetic, relaxed, and fit!

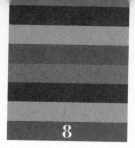

8

Week Four: Step 3: Stress Less and Enjoy

$\mathcal{W}$e all have to deal with stress—it's a part of life and there is no getting around it or rid of it. In fact, some types of stress are actually good for you because they help you put pressure on yourself to complete tasks and get through the day. The problem comes when your stress crosses the line from helping you get stuff done to stopping you from living a happy and productive life.

In this third and final step, we will tackle reducing the stresses that can lead to heart disease. Recognizing and dealing with stress is very different from changing your diet or adding exercise to your life. What one of us may consider stressful someone else might not. Therefore, we're going to explain exactly what stress is, how to tell the good stress from the bad stress, and finally how to help you de-stress your life.

What Is Stress?

We all think we know when we're stressed. We go around telling everyone how stressed we are or we see it in others. But what is it exactly and why is it so bad when we can't get rid of it?

Simply defined, stress is a feeling of emotional or physical tension and is our response to any situation or thing that makes us anxious, fearful, uneasy, or frustrated. Situations in our life we consider difficult or unmanageable also create anxiety and stress. There is another side, though, and sometimes small quantities of stress can motivate us and help us be more productive. However, too much stress can be harmful, setting the stage for poor health and unhealthy behaviors such as overeating, excessive drinking, smoking, and so on. We all feel stress, but we feel it in different amounts and react to it in different ways. Learning to deal with stress in a positive way is essential for our overall heart health.

How Stress Harms Us

For many women, the stress of simply taking care of a home would be enough to drive most men around the bend. The details of running a home are mind-boggling: laundry, ironing, cleaning, paying bills, cooking, shopping, and serving meals. These tasks alone add up to a full-time job. If you have children or an elderly parent to take care of, well, it's no wonder that many women are stressed. Notice that we haven't even talked about holding down a job. Even if you have a partner who shares in these tasks, chances are you are still shouldering most of the responsibility. And if you are taking care of a parent (even if it is his parent), we can practically guarantee that you are the one totally responsible for his or her care. The weaker sex we are not, but we aren't invincible. Yes, we may be able to juggle many responsibilities, but we cannot do it forever without it taking a toll on our health.

Many of our patients tell us that they feel scheduled from the moment they wake up in the morning until they go to sleep at night. As women, we are constantly doing for others and not taking time for ourselves. Many of us don't slow down until we get sick and have no other choice, but even that doesn't mean life suddenly becomes stress free because we are ill. In fact, being sick often creates a situation where if we don't do something, it just doesn't get done, so there's stress involved in trying to get well again as quickly as possible.

If your life resembles this out-of-control merry-go-round, you must find ways to cope better. You can do this by learning how to reduce the stress, because if you don't, the stress will damage both your physical and mental health.

The Stress Factor in Heart Disease

When we're under high levels of stress, our heart beats faster, our blood pressure rises, our blood sugar increases, and we can gain weight. In fact, women tend to store the extra weight gained from stress in their belly.

Medical science still hasn't identified precisely how stress increases the risk of heart disease. It may be that stress is simply a risk factor, or it could be that stress is the catalyst that triggers other risk factors, like high cholesterol, high blood pressure, and gaining weight, or makes them worse because of the tendency to overeat, smoke, drink, or be inactive when we are experiencing stress. What we do know is that stress takes its toll on Black women and Latinas who are already at high risk for heart disease.

We already know that both Latinas and African-American women rank high on the number of risk factors that lead to heart disease because of poor eating habits, smoking, and inactivity—and the irony here is that when we feel stressed, we tend to smoke more, drink more, mope around the house, and overeat! Unless we find a proactive way to manage stress, we can actually cause more health problems that will lead to even more stress in the long run.

The Main Causes of Stress

Stress is not unique to Latinas and African-American women, and there certainly are many members of our community who have learned to manage it. It's not an impossible task. But there is no denying that we do have to deal with cultural sources of stress that do not affect other races. Women of color, on the whole, tend to shoulder more responsibility than women in other cultures, especially in the United States. Stress for Hispanic women comes from being the principal caregiver for their entire family, and for Black women it stems from the fact that many are single mothers. What they have in common is that both of these situations don't have any natural outlet for stress. This means we must learn how to relieve stress before it damages our health. Let's look a bit more in detail at the causes of stress common to women of color.

Hispanic women report many more health-related sources of stress than the general public. Thirty-five percent of Hispanic women consider the health problems of their spouse, partner, parents, or children a significant source of stress versus 24 percent of the general public. These days it's common for women to be taking care of two families: their own kids and husband as well as their aging parents. In the Hispanic community, where the family is so important, the woman, who is already stressed from taking care of everyone, is also the one these same family members turn to help alleviate their stress. Latinas also list job and money as other main sources of stress.

Black women appear to handle stress somewhat differently. White women tend to find stress relief by devoting time to their children or seeking support and friendship from others, called by stress researchers a "tend and befriend" response. Black women, though, tend, befriend, mend, and keep it in. The Black culture in America has evolved in a way different from any other race, and in order for it to thrive the way it has, Black women had to become resourceful and productive, loyal and loving. As Toni Morrison so eloquently put it, we "invented ourselves." The ability to rise against overwhelming odds leads to the concept of the strong Black woman. Unfortunately, this moniker works against us. In our attempt to remain strong, as we are expected to be, we keep our feelings and emotions bottled up while we help everyone else.

These two cultures rely on us women to hold everything and everyone together all the time, but to whom do we turn? And at what cost to our health do we remain the caregiver to all but ourselves?

The Effect of Chronic Stress on the Heart

In our daily lives, we suffer from two types of stressful situations: One type is the crisis that is solved and goes away. The other type doesn't—it's chronic. Chronic stress is the damaging kind that just doesn't ease up. Chronic stress may be caused by having to take care of an ailing family member, not having a job, not making enough money, being overweight, or having other health issues yourself. Whatever the cause, it impacts your heart.

Here is what we know:

- **Stress activates our sympathetic nervous system.** This is the automatic part of our nervous system that affects the running of many organs like the heart and the brain. When stress occurs, the body prepares to take action. This preparation is called the fight-or-flight response. In the fight-or-flight response, levels of many hormones like adrenaline increase significantly with an overall effect of making a lot of stored energy—glucose (sugar) and fat—available to our body so that we can get away from danger.

- **Stress increases the rate at which the heart beats** while causing the arteries to constrict, thereby decreasing blood flow to the heart.

- **Stress leads to an increase in certain factors in the blood,** which can damage the arteries that supply blood and nutrients to the heart, thereby increasing the chances of heart disease.

- **Stress causes the blood to become stickier,** increasing the likelihood of an artery-clogging blood clot, which can lead to a heart attack.

- **Stress stops the body from ridding itself of fat molecules,** raising cholesterol levels, at least temporarily.

- **Stress is often related to weight gain and obesity** because it may influence cravings for salt, fat, and sugar to counteract tension. The stress hormone cortisol is also responsible for the accumulation of abdominal fat and may be the primary connection between stress and weight gain.

- **Stress can complicate existing diabetes.** In people who have diabetes, the fight-or-flight response does not work well. Insulin, which regulates the blood glucose levels, is not always able to let the extra energy into the cells and thus glucose increases in the blood. In addition, the stress hormone cortisol can cause a direct increase in the levels of glucose in the blood.

• **Stress may also lead to depression or anxiety.** Studies suggest that the inability to adapt to stress is associated with the onset of depression or anxiety. In one small study, people who experienced a stressful situation had a much higher chance of developing depression in the months following.

Gauging Your Stress Level

As we've said before, we are all under some level of stress, but how much stress is the key to whether or not it is a problem and contributing to ill health.

Anything that makes you feel stressed is called a stressor. In order to control your stress, you must first identify the stressors in your life so that you can work toward releasing the tension they cause. Stressors can be minor hassles, minor or major lifestyle changes, or a combination of both.

Take a moment to think about your daily activities at work and at home, because any activity has the potential to be stressful. Stress can be caused by a physical or emotional change and any alteration you must make to your daily routine. Granted, some changes are good and you may be stressed for a while until these new activities become routine, but be aware of the stress that doesn't go away.

Common Stressors

- daily hassles (commuting, shopping, cooking, housekeeping, and so on.)
- work overload
- starting a new job
- losing a job
- retiring
- crowds
- illness (yours or that of a family member or friend)
- financial problems
- legal problems
- moving into a new house or apartment
- death of a friend or relative
- ending a romantic relationship
- disagreements with family, friends, or coworkers

Of course, this is a general list of categories and is in no way complete; life is too complicated to be able to list everything that may be a stressor. But this will give you an idea of the range of situations that can cause stress. Think of what is causing your stress and write it in your notebook.

The Warning Signs of Stress

Whenever you are exposed to a stressor for a long period of time, your body reacts to it and gives you warning signals that something is wrong. Bottom line is that there are not enough hours in the day for all the things we have to do and want to do. Unfortunately, being so busy can lead to ignoring these signs. If you ignore them, you aren't giving your body the needed break it so desperately needs to protect itself from developing problems or from making existing medical problems worse. These signs are a real indication that you need to slow down and learn to cope with this stressor to disarm its bad influence on your daily life.

Physical signs may include dizziness, general aches and pains, grinding teeth, clenched jaws, headaches, indigestion, muscle tension, difficulty sleeping, racing heartbeat, ringing in the ears, stooped posture, sweaty palms, tiredness, exhaustion, trembling, weight gain or loss.

Emotional signs may include anxiety, crying, anger, depression, feeling of powerlessness or loneliness, mood swings, irritability, negative thinking, nervousness, sadness.

Mental signs can include inability to concentrate, no sense of humor, forgetfulness or poor memory, constant worrying, difficulty making decisions, or lack of creativity.

Behavioral signs can include overeating or compulsive eating; excessive drinking, smoking, or use of other drugs; bossiness, quick-temperedness, impulsive actions, criticism of others; frequent job changes; withdrawal from personal relationships or social situations.

Getting Stress Under Control

This week you are going to deal with stress in the same positive way you dealt with changing your eating habits and starting an exercise regime. What you learn in this chapter will add the final element of what you need to know to slow down or even prevent heart disease.

Learning to control your stress is different from mastering the first two steps, because stress and the effect it has on you are completely individual. No one around you may know you are stressed. Or the very same stressor can elicit different levels of stress in those around you. Don't feel embarrassed or ashamed if you are stressed by the daily grind but a friend isn't. And don't act as if everything is fine when it's not. Even one stressful situation may be enough to badly influence your health, so if only one or two things stress you out, it's best to deal with them. If you have many stressors in your life, don't despair; there is a way to lessen them once you know how.

Alicia wanted to come to our weekly educational sessions to learn more about her heart health. The difficulty was that it was so stressful for her to make all the arrangements to get to the class. She had to leave work early, rush like a lunatic, make arrangements for her children (although we offered to let them sit in the back and even offered to provide healthy snacks for them), and take a bus to and from the class, and then she worried the entire time about all the things she needed to do at home. We finally had to tell her that we felt she was adding way too much stress to her life to try to learn about stress reduction! She agreed, and together we came up with other options that were available to her and much less stressful. We actually shared a good laugh about it too.

If you feel overwhelmed by your list of stressors, seeking professional help can put you on the right track in dealing with stress in your life. Licensed social workers, psychologists, and psychiatrists can teach you stress-management strategies, including relaxation techniques. Support groups of various types are also available through the community, in places of worship, or in hospitals and are very useful in helping you adjust your attitude to decrease daily stress.

While it is impossible to live your life completely stress free, it is possible to reduce the harmful effects of certain stressors. Remember that small steps make a difference— so removing even one or two items from your list will make a significant difference in how you feel, on what you do, and ultimately on your overall health.

Stress-Reduction Techniques

In order to cope with stress, you need to learn how to relax. Relaxing is a learned skill—it takes commitment and practice. It is more than sitting back and being quiet. Rather, it's an active process involving techniques that calm your body and mind. True relaxation requires becoming sensitive to your basic needs for peace, self-awareness, and thoughtful reflection. The challenge is being willing to meet these needs rather than dismissing them.

Listed below are a number of effective relaxation methods. When you find one that works for you, practice it every day for at least thirty minutes. Taking the time to practice simple relaxation techniques gives you the chance to unwind and get ready for life's next challenge.

Deep Breathing

Most people figure they know how to breathe—they've been doing it since birth! But in fact, most of us breathe far too shallowly, from the stomach instead of the diaphragm. During diaphragmatic ("deep") breathing, each breath is smooth, even, and rhythmic. Diaphragmatic breathing eases the intake of oxygen and the elimination of carbon dioxide (one of the body's waste products) with the least amount of effort.

You probably rely on your chest instead of your diaphragm to fill your lungs with air. This is called chest breathing, and it stimulates a network of nerves that control your heart, stomach, and intestines. An important job of your nervous system is to regulate digestion and the muscle contractions that eliminate solid waste. So when you breathe from your chest, it activates the parts of your nervous system that produce many uncomfortable sensations experienced during periods of stress. Chest breathing also supplies the muscles with more oxygen to fuel the cells in the body, preparing you to fight or flee.

Deep breathing, on the other hand, triggers the part of the nervous system that stops the fight-or-flight response. This is why you can't be physically relaxed and stressed at the same time. With deep breathing, there's a good mix of oxygen coming into the lungs and carbon dioxide going out, and the fight-or-flight system comes to a screeching halt. Deep breathing also releases the body's own painkillers so you'll feel more comfortable. Learning how to breathe deeply is an important step in managing stress.

Controlled Breathing Step by Step

Step 1. Find a quiet, comfortable place. Close your eyes so you won't be distracted.

Step 2. Place one hand above your belly button and the other on your chest. Observe how you breathe. Notice which hand rises more as you inhale. If you're trying for deep breathing, your belly will push out and lift your bottom hand during the inhalation phase, while your top hand will rest rock still on your chest. (It's okay to look fat!) If your belly doesn't move or moves less than your chest, then you're breathing from your chest and your top hand will rise with each breath. You can easily correct the way you have been breathing.

Step 3. Draw a normal amount of air deep into the bottom of your lungs. Every time you breathe in this way, your abdomen expands. When you breathe out, your abdomen is sucked back in. Imagine that you're blowing up a large balloon inside your belly.

Step 4. Inhale slowly and deeply, drawing air deeply into your lungs to inflate your abdomen. Some people prefer to breathe in through their nose and out through their mouth. Don't let the air out all at once; allow the air to flow evenly as you breathe in and out.

Step 5. Count "1" silently as you breathe in. As you breathe out, picture the word "relax" or any focus word or words (such as "let go") or image that conveys a calm, relaxed state as you relax. Count "2" when you breathe in and picture your focus word when you breathe out. Count up to 10 and then go back to the beginning and count again.

Breathe Your Way to Relaxation

Now that you've learned how to breathe correctly from your diaphragm, you can start practicing this breathing exercise.

Find a comfortable, quiet location and close your eyes.

Mentally count "1" as you breathe in, relax as you breathe out. Gently exhale as if you were trying to flicker the flame of a candle without extinguishing it, or blow across a spoonful of soup without spilling.

As you breathe in, push your belly out; as you exhale, draw your belly in. Keep your chest still throughout.

Focus your attention on the number or relaxing word without letting other thoughts cross your mind. Maintain a comfortable rate of breathing that is even and smooth.

Count up to 10 and repeat.

PROGRESSIVE MUSCLE RELAXATION

Switch your thoughts to yourself and your breathing. Take a few deep breaths, exhaling slowly. Mentally scan your body. Notice areas that feel tense or cramped. Loosen up these areas. Let go of as much tension as you can. Rotate your head in a smooth, circular motion once or twice. (Stop any movements that cause pain!) Roll your shoulders forward and backward several times. Let all of your muscles completely relax. Recall a pleasant thought for a few seconds. Take another deep breath and exhale slowly. You should feel relaxed.

MENTAL IMAGERY RELAXATION

Mental imagery relaxation, or guided imagery, is a form of focused relaxation that helps create harmony between the mind and body. Guided imagery coaches you in creating calm, peaceful images in your mind—a "mental escape." Identify your self-talk, that is, what you are saying to yourself about what is going on with your illness or situation. It is important to identify negative self-talk and develop healthy, positive self-talk. By making affirmations, you can counteract negative thoughts and emotions.

MUSIC RELAXATION

Combine relaxation exercises with your favorite music. Select the type of music that lifts your mood or that you find soothing or calming. Some people find it easier to relax while listening to specially designed relaxation audiotapes, which provide music and relaxation instructions.

BIOFEEDBACK

Biofeedback helps you learn stress-reduction skills by using various instruments to measure temperature, heart rate, muscle tension, and other vital signs as you attempt to relax. The goal of biofeedback is to teach you to monitor your own body as you relax. It helps you gain control over certain bodily functions that cause tension and physical pain. If a headache, such as a migraine, begins slowly, many people can use biofeedback to stop the attack before it becomes full-blown.

Meditation

Mediation can help reduce the severity of congestive heart failure. Researchers at the University of Pennsylvania discovered that patients who meditated had significant improvement on a six-minute walk test compared to the nonmeditation group, as well as fewer rehospitalizations. With the technique we describe below, you'll be able to relax in situations causing tension even in the middle of a busy day, giving you lots more control over how your body reacts to stress. When you find yourself getting tense at work or home, rather than allowing stress to build up, use the first signs of tension or anxiety feelings as a cue to start a relaxation technique.

How to Meditate

1. Sit or lie down and close your eyes.
2. Start at the top of your head and slowly relax each group of muscles, one by one: scalp, neck, left arm and hand, right arm and hand, back, waist, left side of body, right side of body, and so on.
3. When all of your muscles are totally relaxed, begin counting slowly, from 1 to 5. As you mentally say the number 1, imagine yourself either walking down stairs, descending an escalator, or floating in a balloon, feeling more deeply relaxed. With each number, you feel yourself becoming more and more deeply relaxed.

   As you count, keep imagining yourself descending into a state of deeper and deeper relaxation. After every number, you will find yourself becoming more and more deeply relaxed until you reach 5, when you will feel completely relaxed.

   Don't rush the countdown. Wait to go to the next number until you're really relaxing. As you count down, you will feel yourself more deeply relaxed.
4. Now move out of the relaxation period, counting from 5 to 1. On the count of 5, you can move your legs and feet. On the count of 4, you can move your arms and hands. On the count of 3, you can move your torso. On the count of 2, you can move your head and neck. On the count of 1, gently open your eyes and you'll feel completely relaxed.

Visualization

As your body relaxes, so does your brain, and as your brain relaxes, so does your body. One way to deepen your feelings of relaxation is through visualization.

Athletes use visualization to rehearse their moves before going into action. World-class skiers imagine themselves negotiating every inch of a hairpin turn on a ski slope, hockey players picture where they want to shoot a puck, and gymnasts visualize their moves as much in their mind's eye as in actual practice. Medical patients can use the same visualization skills to control physical tension that aggravates symptoms. Because the body does not distinguish between an event that occurs in the here and now and one that is imagined, what we visualize can affect our body as much as a real experience.

When you do a visualization relaxation exercise, you're basically creating a word, phrase, or mental image.

How to Visualize

The key to effective visualizing is calling to mind a nice, safe, pleasant place. The more clearly you can bring this place to mind—including details of sights, sounds, textures, and smells—the deeper your relaxation experience.

Close your eyes. Imagine a nice, safe, pleasant place. Fill in all the details that would surround you in this place. For example, many people find that lying in a meadow on a mountainside is a relaxing scene that they can easily call up. Don't think of a simple snapshot—involve all of your senses to create what the mountain area really looks like. Hear the sweet brook flowing beside you, smell the green grass, and feel the cool breeze brushing your cheeks. Hear the playful calls of the birds in the distance. Feel the warmth of the sun on your head, your chest, your legs, and the soft sleeping bag you're lying on. Let all of your senses transport you to this image.

Many people find lying on a beach a relaxing scene that they can easily incorporate into their relaxation exercises. Again, don't simply recall a "snapshot" of the ocean. Get all of your senses involved to create what an ocean scene is really like. Smell the salty spray of ocean mist in the air and feel the wind blowing in your hair. Hear the playful cries of the seagulls, the crashing of waves rolling rhythmically onto the shore. Feel the warmth of the sun on your head, your chest, your legs, and the soft towel you're lying on, warmed by the soft white sand. Imagine the white, soft, puffy clouds floating against a deep blue sky. Engage all of your senses to transport you to this image.

Of course, if you have a fear of water, this would not be relaxing to you. Choose something that does not elicit fear or anxiety, such as being on a snowy mountaintop. We all have places that are special to us where we feel relaxed and at peace. Whether it's a bench in your favorite park, a lakeside, or a special chair or room in your own home, it will be unique to you and your experiences.

Just as learning how to breathe relaxes your body, learning to put your brain through its paces with visualization can help you relax. It doesn't matter what you visualize. What matters is being able to take a brief mental trip to your favorite or special place and experience a sense of peace and renewal.

Six Steps for Controlling Stress

1. Identify everything you need to do in your daily life for the coming week and make a list.

Think of this as your to-do list and don't let the number of duties on your list cause you even more stress. If you find that you are overwhelmed by the number of things you must do in a week, then start by taking it one day at a time. The purpose of this list is to let you see what you can control and what you cannot control. So look at your list and cross off everything that you cannot control. Leave these things behind and take responsibility for and control only what you can. When you get used to the idea that you can (and must) eliminate some of your duties to reduce your stress, then you can start thinking in terms of weeks. Again, if you find you can't manage the stress in your life, seek out professional help.

Wait a day and then look at your list again. We're betting that you, like the rest of us, have lots of things to accomplish and not enough time to do them. Decide which listed jobs or activities are not essential. Cross off anything you can live without doing. Don't just cross off the stuff you don't want to do or don't necessarily like to do, like exercising. Remember that you are eliminating the tasks that are not essential to your quality of life (and exercising is essential).

PRIORITIZE AND DELEGATE

Prioritize the tasks that are left on your list in their order of importance. Next, see what you must do yourself and what you can ask family, friends, and coworkers to help you do. Yes, there is help available to all of us; we just have to know whom we can count on to help us. Some of us never considered this an option—it's time to change that.

For instance, if you always walk your child to and from school, maybe you can share this job with a classmate's parent (or better, the parents of several classmates). Meet with them and see if you can work out an arrangement where you alternate weeks, or you take the kids to school and the other parent picks them up. The other parents will also welcome the free time this provides.

When we say delegate, we do not mean ask someone else to do your work for you, but we do want you to think a little outside the box and your comfort zone. You may be worrying about what others may think if you don't take and pick up your kids every day. Don't stress yourself out with these thoughts and the feeling of selfishness or guilt they may bring about. There is no room for these feelings, because they can quickly turn into anger and that's not healthy for you or your family. You are not only allowed some alone time or some downtime, you need time alone and to slow down. It's okay to ask for help, so go through the list and see what can be delegated, shared, or postponed, and then prioritize the remaining tasks. We bet that your list is looking more manageable already.

Don't forget that small steps—even removing only one or two tasks from your to-do list—will make a significant difference in how you feel, what you do, and ultimately your overall health.

SCHEDULE "YOU" TIME

Now that you have pared down your to-do list to what is absolutely necessary, you should be able to find some time for yourself. The first thing you need to do is go through your calendar and see exactly what time you do have. Is there now a free morning, afternoon, or evening during the week? Think of what you'd like to do during that time. It can be as simple as taking a long bath, calling a friend on the phone, or meeting a friend for breakfast, lunch, or dinner. Maybe there's time for a knitting or exercise class, a movie, or a walk in the park. The point is that it doesn't matter as long as it is something you enjoy and that it's a break from your regular routine. Block out this time as if it is an important appointment (because it is) or think of it as a "prescription" for health from your doctor.

Prepare for this special time. For example, if you've chosen to knit every Thursday at 11 A.M., then by Wednesday evening be certain that you have yarn, a pattern, and the right size needles. After all, if your son had a baseball practice on Thursdays at 11 A.M., you'd be certain by Wednesday evening that his uniform was clean, and his bat, hat, glove, and water bottle were in the duffel bag, wouldn't you? Take the time to prepare for your activity in the same way—it is just as important!

ORGANIZE YOUR LIVING SPACE

A cluttered and disorganized home can literally drain your energy and cause additional stress! Just think of the anxiety you feel when you can't find something in a hurry. It causes stress and wastes precious time that you could be using for something more productive. If you declutter your home, get organized about cleaning (don't hesitate to enlist family members to help or, at least, clean up after themselves), and keep ahead of that laundry pile and the dirty dishes, you will create a soothing environment that can be a haven where you can escape from the stressors in your life.

ORGANIZE YOUR TIME

Make and stick to a schedule and learn to say no to excessive demands on your time. Also be realistic and flexible when you plan your schedule. Be creative and think of shortcuts to make tasks go faster. Do the important jobs first and leave the less important ones for later. Don't get into the habit of killing time with lots of small and insignificant things so that you're too tired or don't have enough time to do the things that count. Organize your time and you'll be less frantic and have more time for the things that energize and de-stress you.

DEVELOP A SUPPORTIVE CIRCLE

Learn to share your troubles. As we know, Black women and Latinas tend to bottle everything inside. This isn't because we want to—this behavior has evolved over time in our cultures. We have to appear strong in order to help those around us, but the truth is that we need to share what is bothering us, too. We need to unload our problems before they fester inside and destroy our health.

Sharing your troubles will not make you appear weak, because whomever you confide in probably has problems that you can help with. You're not necessarily looking for advice, though; you need someone who cares about you to listen. It's a fact that women who have a supportive social circle, a close friend or two, or a partner who listens in times of crisis enjoy healthier, less stressful lives—and they have more fun. Very often just by knowing that you are not alone in dealing with the stress of everyday life and hearing from other women how they deal with stress can help reduce your own daily anxieties. If you make the commitment to meet more people, and develop close relationships with those you trust, you'll reap this benefit.

GET A HOBBY

We're sure you have things you've always wanted to do or try, and now that you've scheduled the time, get out there and enjoy a hobby. Hobbies are fun. Even simple hobbies like drawing, playing cards, doing crossword puzzles or sudoku, and gardening are great stress relievers, plus they help you stay in touch with your creative side.

2. Have a Positive Attitude and Good Self-Esteem

A positive attitude and good self-esteem help you view stress as a challenge rather than a problem. A positive attitude keeps you in control when there are inevitable changes in your life. With a positive attitude, you believe that you have the ability to improve certain situations and have the courage to admit when there's nothing you can do to change what's going on.

The following tips will help you maintain a positive attitude during stressful situations or when you need to prepare yourself for a potentially stressful situation:

- Stay calm. Stop what you're doing. Breathe deeply. Reflect on your choices.

- Tell yourself you can get through this situation.
- Remain objective, realistic, and flexible.
- Keep the situation in perspective. Think about the possible solutions. Choose one that is the most acceptable and feasible.
- Prepare for the worst possible outcome—but know that odds are it will never be as bad as you imagined.
- Know that you can always learn something from every situation.

3. Start the Day on a Healthy Note

Here are some healthy lifestyle habits to incorporate into your morning routine that will better prepare you to handle everyday stress. Experiment with one, several, or all, or add your own until you find what suits you and what works best.

ADD MUSIC

Listening to music reduces stress and has a positive effect on mental and physical health. Turn on the radio, put on your favorite CD, or listen to your MP3 player as part of your morning routine to start your day with positive energy. Music also complements other healthy lifestyle habits by adding a sense of peace, putting a spring in your step on a morning walk, or stimulating your mind as you write in your journal.

STRETCH IN THE SHOWER

Hot water loosens up the muscles, so it's easier to get a good stretch. The act of stretching also releases the stored tension we hold in our muscles and enables us to start the day feeling more relaxed, at peace, and ready to handle whatever comes our way.

EAT A BALANCED BREAKFAST

At the risk of sounding like your mother, it really is true that breakfast is the most important meal of the day. A healthy, well-balanced meal of protein, whole grain (or complex carb) and fruit in the morning can maintain your blood sugar levels to give you the sustenance you need to think clearly so you can handle physical and mental stress. Coffee is fine, but forget the doughnut. If you sometimes need to eat on the run, skip the doughnut and substitute oatmeal, granola, a piece of fruit or a low-fat yogurt drink. When you can, get up early enough to sit down and eat your breakfast. This action will also help to set the tone for your day.

4. Rediscover the Art of Relaxation

You are going to reacquaint your new self with your old friend relaxation, and you'll be surprised how easy it is. If you have trouble remembering how to relax (or maybe you never really learned) here's what to do.

THINK OF ACTIVITIES THAT HAVE HELPED YOU RELAX IN THE PAST

Maybe you had a favorite hobby or played an instrument or danced. If nothing comes to mind, then think of enjoyable past experiences and activities that hold pleasant memories, memories that put a smile on your face. Jot these down in your journal and see if you can integrate them into your daily life.

IMAGINE YOUR PERFECT DAY

If you had a free day without a care in the world, what would you do? Write it down. This is huge, because acknowledging it and writing it down make it real and attainable. Take as long as you need and give this exercise the serious thought that it deserves. Naming it is a big first step toward attaining it.

RELAX

Relaxing is a learned skill that takes commitment and practice. Relaxation is more than sitting back and being quiet. Rather, it's an active process involving techniques that calm your body and mind. True relaxation requires becoming sensitive to your basic needs for peace, self-awareness, and thoughtful reflection. The challenge is being willing to meet these needs rather than dismissing

them. See pages 121–122 for various ways to integrate relaxation into your life.

5. Get Enough Sleep

You cannot fight stress or cope effectively with what life
throws at you without proper rest. During sleep, your body
recovers from physical problems and stressful events. At
least eight hours of sleep is critical, and some of us need
even more. Naps work for some people to recharge those
batteries during the day. When your body needs rest, it lets
you know—don't ignore the signs. Make sure that the time
you spend resting is long enough so you wake refreshed.

If you have trouble sleeping, here are some suggestions:

- Establish a regular sleep schedule. Go to bed and get up at the same time every day, including weekends.
- Make sure your bed and surroundings are comfortable. Arrange the pillows so you can maintain a comfortable position.
- Keep your bedroom dark and quiet (use an eyeshade or ear plugs).
- Use your bedroom only for sleeping and sex; move the TV or the computer to another room.
- Avoid naps if they interfere with your sleeping through the night.
- Get your troubles off your mind. You won't be able to sleep if you are nervous or anxious.
- Listen to relaxing music to lull you off to sleep.
- Do *not* take over-the-counter sleeping aids or borrow some

from your friends or family. Not only can some sleep medications interfere with other medications you are taking, some can leave you feeling foggy the next day. There are a number of new sleep medications on the market and if you really need to take something, speak with your doctor.

- If you can't sleep, get up and out of bed and do something relaxing—read a book, watch TV, and so on—until you feel tired.
- Avoid drinking caffeine anytime after breakfast. This doesn't mean just coffee; watch those soft drinks and iced teas you drink for lunch, dinner, and in between because many contain caffeine.

6. Enjoy Your Friends and Family

Family gatherings or meeting with friends can be great fun. Once you learn to schedule so that you have some free time, take advantage of it to be with those you love and care about. Family activities can range from playing board or computer games to watching movies, singing, going for walks, bowling, playing cards, or Sunday dinner. The activity doesn't matter. Simply doing the things we love and enjoying time with people we love goes a long way to making for a stress-free life.

As you've seen, you don't have to spend money or make major life changes. Small steps make such a big difference in improving quality of life.

When you complete week four, reward yourself. Choose something special to celebrate any of your small accomplishments. Treat yourself to something that you have always wanted. Take a night off and go to the movies and dinner with your girlfriends.

While you're in this great mood, plan the rest of the month in your journal to ensure you continue to do the things that will make you happy and less stressed. Congratulations on your progress.

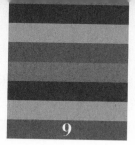

9

Week Five: FEAST: Putting It All Together for the Rest of Your Life!

*P*atricia is the single mother of two boys: André, age ten, and Wayne, six. Because of working a full-time job, household chores, her sons' sports and schoolwork, her life seemed overwhelming. Her boys were always clamoring to stop for fast food after practice, and her freezer was filled with microwavable convenience foods. Her lifestyle started to take its toll. Patricia was tired, depressed, and exhausted. She felt that she had no time to relax and nothing to look forward to—she was in a vicious cycle.

At her recent doctor's visit, she learned that her cholesterol and blood pressure were up and her diabetes was out of control. She was referred for a stress test due to her high blood pressure and vague symptoms of extreme fatigue, shortness of breath, and occasional palpitations in her chest. With our suggestions, she was able to make a number of small changes, including limiting the fast-food stops to once a week and making time to cook real meals, at least on Sunday when the entire family sat down together to eat—without watching TV.

It was a start, and to everyone's surprise, it was also fun. This time together with her family allowed Patricia to begin to relax and enjoy her kids so she was able to talk to them instead of yelling all the time. The family also began to take turns picking what to do on Saturday afternoons and then would end their day together snuggling up with a movie. Patricia was healthier and happier because she was less stressed and eating better, and her new lifestyle set a great example for her boys too.

Patricia's example shows you that it is possible to make small changes to your life, even if you have a job and a family. The changes you must make are not drastic. They are small, but they are crucial to getting you on the road to health. You don't have to make all the changes at once. You can make these changes gradually, but you do have to change. Once you start seeing the benefits (and you will), you'll have no trouble sticking to your new habits. Like Patricia, your simple small steps will help you to arrive at a healthier lifestyle.

When we make changes in our lives through new behaviors, we can make them permanent only if they become habits. Enthusiasm can get you started, but enthusiasm alone is not enough to maintain a change in long-term behavior. You must turn enthusiasm for doing something new into a habit so that you just do it without thinking. When this happens and you develop new healthy habits, you've made it. You have become heart smart!

It is now time to celebrate all the small steps that you have accomplished throughout the past four weeks and to make the heart-smart commitment for the rest of your life. Week five is the time to review where you were successful, but even more important is to review where you failed. It's important to celebrate your successes and be proud of them. But you will undoubtedly learn a lot from your failures. It's like when you were a kid and you made a mistake at school and had to do your project over or rewrite something several times as a homework (or detention) assignment. We bet you never forgot what subject it was, the teacher's name, or the grade you received. It's not necessary to punish yourself, but looking at what didn't work can help you determine different choices that will help you to change.

Looking back over the past three weeks, think about your strengths and weaknesses and record them in your notebook. Did you have a harder time with eating than with exercise or managing stress? Was it easy for you to choose to eat healthier food? As you moved on to step two and added exercise, maybe you did great with the exercise but couldn't maintain the healthier eating. Don't worry, it's common for one aspect of the program to work better than another when taking on so many new lifestyle changes over a fairly short period of time.

Don't be discouraged. Even if you feel that you took three steps forward and one back, read what you wrote in your journal to remind you how you felt in the weeks when you struggled. Then think about why this may have happened. Read about how others reacted to your changes. Did they support your changes or try to sabotage them? Did that contribute to a success or a failure? Why? Your faithful recording of this time will help you to understand yourself better and see what motivates you. Now let's put this all together and make the commitment for life!

FEAST: Putting It All Together

You need to FEAST in order to make this plan a success and to be able to stick to it. You'll be able to make these changes. If you're motivated enough to have read this far, we're sure you're already thinking of the future. Don't be discouraged, though, even if you slip occasionally and revert back to your old habits. The key to success is being able to pick yourself up and get back on the road to health. The longer you live your new lifestyle, the easier it will be and the less you'll slide back to your unhealthy past. This chapter will show you how to stay on that track and how to handle the occasional slip by using the acronym FEAST:

Family and Friends

Women who enlist the help or support of their partner or are part of a group are the ones most likely to stay motivated and succeed in achieving their goals. This means that the more people you reach out to—family, friends, neighbors, church members—the more likely you are to make the changes necessary for total heart health. Of course they won't be with you every time you choose to eat an apple instead of a piece of cake, or decide to cook instead of stopping for fast food, or watch you exercise. Instead, let people know that you are making positive changes in your life. If they are aware of what you're doing, they can encourage you or compliment you on your achievements. Or you may be lucky enough to have friends or family who will go on regular walks with you or who will follow your example and adopt the rules for healthy cooking (especially at holidays and family gatherings). By reaching out to others you not only ensure your success; you impart valuable knowledge to others, especially when they start seeing the results of a healthier, fit you.

First, decide what kind of support you need and then reach out to the people you feel will be the most supportive. Think of those you trust. Which person is best suited to give you positive reinforcement or even join you? If you're the independent type that can stay focused and is goal oriented, that's great, but if you're not, enlist help.

Remember to log your achievements in your journal. After a couple of weeks, be sure to reread your early entries to see how far you've come. Nothing motivates like success! When you do reach special milestones, like a good blood pressure reading, stable blood sugar numbers, lower cholesterol level, or even losing a pound or two, reward yourself. You deserve it.

Eat Healthy

What and how much you eat are important. Heart-healthy food habits can help you reduce at least three of the major risk factors for heart attack: high blood cholesterol, high blood pressure, and excess body weight.

It's okay to snack. Just be sure to choose foods that taste great and are good for you. It's just as easy to buy a piece of fresh fruit as a candy bar. Many produce stores sell carrot and celery sticks. A handful of raw almonds or walnuts or a nonfat yogurt also works. So instead of a bag of chips, pick up a bottle of water and a fresh-food snack. If heart-healthy eating and planning don't come naturally to you, don't be discouraged. Talk to friends, coworkers, or your doctor to help you out and give you suggestions. Even though changing your eating habits may seem overwhelming at first (especially with the other changes you might have to make), trust us, they will become easier as time goes on, especially once you start seeing and feeling the results. Also, you can go back and reread the earlier chapters of this book if you need more reinforcement about why you're changing your life.

Active Lifestyle

All physical activities make a difference to your overall health. Don't think of physical activity in terms of formal exercise, because any moving you do—dancing, swimming, bicycling, household activities, sweeping, vacuuming, raking the leaves, gardening, painting, bowling, mopping, mowing the lawn—contributes to a healthier heart.

Get up and get moving. Otherwise you will continue to have a major risk factor for cardiovascular disease. The more active you are, the better. Consider the fact that most women become less active during their teenage years and then tend to stay less physically active than men for the rest of their lives.

Regular physical activity helps reduce your risk of heart disease by helping to lower blood pressure; controlling blood cholesterol, diabetes, and obesity; building stronger bones; helping to reduce anxiety and depression; and increasing your energy levels. Being physically active also increases self-esteem because not only will you feel better, you'll look better too! Be active every day!

To make physical activity a regular part of your daily routine, keep track in your journal of how active you are. Include everything you do, such as walking up and down the stairs at home or at work, walking, shopping, housework, or exercise classes. Then, as you did with changes you made in your eating habits, after a few weeks, go back and read your journal to see if you've increased your physical activity and how. If you're now more active than before, again reward yourself.

Keep a log to record your activities and help keep you motivated. Wear comfortable clothes and sneakers or flat shoes with laces. Start slowly. Gradually build up to thirty minutes of activity on most or all days of the week (or whatever your doctor recommends). If you don't have a thirty-minute block of time, you can do ten-minute sessions to meet your goal. Exercise at the same time of day so it becomes a regular part of your lifestyle. For example, you might walk every Monday, Wednesday, Friday, and Saturday from noon to 12:15 or 12:30. Note your activities on a calendar or in a log. Write down the distance or number of steps or length of time of your activity and how you feel after each session. If you miss a day, plan a makeup day or add ten to fifteen minutes to your next session if possible.

Use a variety of activities to maintain your interest and keep from getting bored. Walk one day, swim the next time, then go for a bike ride on the weekend. Join an exercise group, health club, or the Y. Many churches and senior centers offer exercise programs too. (Remember to get your doctor's permission first.) Don't get discouraged if you stop for a while. Get started again gradually and work up to your old pace. Use music to keep you entertained.

Stress Reduction

Although you can't eliminate all of your stress, knowing how to manage it is the next best thing. In order to do this, it helps to keep a positive, glass-is-half-full attitude.

A positive attitude and self-esteem are the best defenses against stress because they help you view stress as a challenge rather than a problem. Make sure you practice the stress-reduction techniques we presented in Chapter 8. Every time something threatens to overwhelm you, keep cool. It's not worth raising your blood pressure. Think it through and come to a conclusion—either you can change a bad situation or you cannot. Just know the difference and know you made the right choice, even if it means walking away. Your health depends on it.

Music brings great health and stress-relief benefits. One of the bonuses of music is that it can be used while you conduct your regular activities so that it really doesn't take time away from your regular schedule.

Once you find a relaxation method that works for you, practice it every day for at least ten minutes. Taking the time to practice simple relaxation techniques gives you the chance to unwind and get ready for life's next challenge.

Take Control of Your Life!

You have taken control of your life. You are learning to eat well, exercise, and reduce stress. Therefore, you must celebrate your accomplishments, make a commitment to lifelong health, and know that even small steps make a difference. When you start doing these three things, you will realize how easy it is to maintain a healthy lifestyle.

Keep your journal for as long as necessary. Maybe you'll want to do it for the rest of your life, or maybe after a period of time these healthy habits will be so ingrained that you do them naturally. Whatever you do, though, make it a point to check in with yourself. Make a list of the steps you're going to take, then put a reminder on your calendar to review each month how you're doing.

Remember that in the first couple of months, it's important that you record all of your daily activities—eating, exercise, and stress reduction—in your log. This way you can see if you met or even exceeded your goals. There will be times when you'll stumble and fall back into old habits. Your journal can help you by pointing out your weaknesses too. It will help you make continued progress. Use it and learn from it. It's an indispensable tool if you use it well.

Part 3

Preventing Heart Disease for a Lifetime

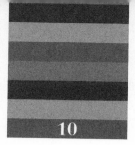

10

The Power of Partnering with Your Doctor

*Y*ou've now been working very hard to get your health on track and have probably enlisted your family, friends, and coworkers to help you succeed. Who else can you involve in your quest to stay healthy and free of heart disease? We want you to think of your doctor as your partner in health.

Just as you prepared for each of the other lifestyle changes, we want you to get into the mind-set of scheduling a yearly checkup. If you have anxiety about going to the doctor for any reason, we will help you put your fears to rest—yearly checkups are vital to your health because they can validate that your lifestyle changes are paying off and they can diagnose potential problems before they become too serious. It doesn't matter if you feel healthy or sick, you should schedule an annual physical checkup.

The Well-Patient Appointment

You probably go to the doctor only when you're sick. We want you to change that way of thinking right now, even though you don't think you have the time or the money to go to the doctor when you're feeling fine. Heart disease is called the "silent killer" for good reason: Many people who suffer fatal heart attacks did not know they had heart disease until it was too late. The best way to diagnose and treat potential heart problems is by seeing your doctor regularly, even when you feel fine.

When your children were little, you took them to see the doctor many times to make sure everything was fine in their development and so that they could get their vaccinations. We bet that if you have dogs or cats, you do the same for them. Well, now it's your turn to make sure that everything is fine or to get early treatment if it's not.

You've already made the major lifestyle changes necessary to keep your heart healthy, but what if something more serious is going on? You want to know so that you can get it corrected before you get sick. Preventative medicine is something we have all learned to live with. We get mammograms and Pap smears yearly, we go to the dentist for checkups and cleanings every year, so why not the medical doctor or internist? These visits are crucial to your health, both to prevent future problems and for early detection of heart disease, especially for women of color.

If you do not have health insurance and the cost of the doctor is keeping you from making an appointment, there are other avenues available to you that can ease the burden of health-care costs. Appendix B lists various agencies/centers along with how to contact them. We've listed prescription assistance information as well, so check it out.

Finding a Doctor

If you do not have a family doctor, now is the time to get one. But knowing where to start isn't that easy these days.

- Ask friends, family members, or coworkers if they have a personal doctor they like a lot. Chances are if someone you know likes her doctor, you'll like this doctor too.
- Get a list of participating physicians in your health insurance plan and check if any of the physicians are on your recommended list.
- Talk to your coworkers who have the same insurance plan as you and ask for the name of their doctor. Also ask if they had a negative experience with any doctor on the plan and why.
- Call your local hospital and ask if they can provide of a list of doctors who accept your insurance. Some hospitals have a Web site with a listing of physicians by name and specialty.
- Choose physicians who are board certified in their specialty— family medicine or general internal medicine. This means they have passed special training and testing in their field.

- Look for a physician with hours and a location convenient to you; otherwise it will be difficult to go even once a year.
- Make sure the physician accepts your insurance. If you do not have insurance, make this clear at the time you make your appointment (and jot down the name of the person you spoke to about this).
- Find a physician who speaks your native tongue or who will provide an interpreter.
- Don't choose a female physician if you'll be comfortable only with a male physician, and vice versa.
- Never use the emergency room for routine appointments, even if that is what you are used to doing. Emergency rooms are for emergencies only. You need a family doctor who can get to know you and your health history.

Take your time and do your homework. This is an important decision, so spend as much time, or more than you would spend researching a car or a computer. After all, you're looking for a doctor to help guide you and your family in making some very important decisions. We want you to find the doctor who will be your partner for a very long time.

The First Visit

You've chosen your doctor and made your appointment. For the first appointment you might want to bring along your spouse or your brother or sister so that you have a second set of ears to listen and take notes. Always ask the doctor to repeat anything you do not understand. Leave the kids at home, if possible.

Be aware that it's not uncommon for an office visit to last only fifteen minutes, so here are some things you can do to be prepared to get the most out of that time.

- Show up on time or a few minutes early.
- Have your insurance cards and medical information handy. If you don't have insurance, make sure you have the name of the person you spoke to when you made the appointment.
- Make a special section in your notebook/journal to keep track of your medical history and bring it with you to the appointment. Be sure to have the following information recorded:
  - A detailed list of all the medications you take (this includes botanicals, vitamins, minerals, aspirin, cold remedies, and allergy medications). Better yet, gather up all the bottles and put them in a bag and bring them with you.
  - Your family history with a listing of the illnesses that affected your parents, grandparents, aunts, uncles, or siblings. Also make a list of any relatives who have died and their cause of death.
- Devote a page to allergies and list all that you have, including those to drugs, food, animals, pollen, and so on.
- Jot down, in detail, any medical complaints you have been having and for how long. Describe the pain or the problem in the way you are feeling it. For example, "I've been getting a stabbing pain in my right arm that moves down from my shoulder to my elbow."
- Make a list of any questions you want to ask the doctor and be

sure to do that at the close of your visit. Just tell the doctor you
have a few questions and then turn to the page in your notebook so you don't forget anything.

During your appointment, make sure you do the following:

- Tell the doctor if you're feeling fine.
- If you do have any complaints, consult your journal and tell the
  doctor about each of them in detail.
- Use your notebook to record anything the doctor says that you
  do not want to forget and don't be afraid to speak up and ask
  that the answer be repeated. There is nothing wrong with po-
  litely asking that the information be repeated if you explain that
  you didn't hear or understand it the first time.

What You Need to Take Away from Your Annual Checkup

Think of your annual doctor's visit as maintenance. Just as
you take your car to get serviced regularly, you are here to
get checked out to make sure you head off any potential
problems. Therefore, at the end of your exam, ask what
you need to do to stay in good health until your next visit.
Use this time to establish a back-and-forth communication
with your doctor. Before you leave the office, you should
ask questions so you know the following:

- Details about your main health problem. What is it called? How serious is it? What are the reasons for it? What do you need to do about it?

- What happens if you cannot comply with all aspects of treatment? Listen to what the doctor tells you, and if you know in your heart you cannot or will not do what is asked, you need to be honest. For example, if your doctor discusses a three-month trial of a weight-loss program to lose ten pounds to help control your blood pressure instead of taking blood pressure medication, be honest about your ability to change your eating habits and stick to an exercise regimen. Unless you are up front with your doctor, he or she will assume that you're following the prescribed orders.

- If there is anything you have been doing that is helping or worsening your problem? Can you continue to exercise, or should you have a stress test before you can continue, or should you be doing more of a workout?

- If medication is prescribed, ask if it can interact with anything you are already taking, how long you'll have to take it, the possible side effects or food interactions.

- What is your risk of heart disease based on your test results (cholesterol, glucose, blood pressure, triglycerides, and weight)?

- When to schedule your next visit, your follow-up blood tests, and how often you'll need to do this.

- What happens if you start feeling sick or if you think you're having a reaction to the medications? Do you call the doctor or go to the emergency room?

- Can your doctor recommend any programs for you to help you accomplish your goals—losing weight, stopping smoking, reducing stress, or learning to prepare meals in a healthier way.

- Request patient educational information. Often doctors have printed brochures that describe medications, illnesses, or treatments. Having a resource you can refer to when you get home will help you to remember and understand what you learned during your visit.

- Ask if there is a nurse or a physician's assistant in the office whom you can call with simple questions.

The Road to Health

You need to have a trusting relationship with your doctor. If you simply don't like the doctor or you don't feel comfortable, then find another one. Sometimes people just don't hit it off and it's not anyone's fault. You need to believe that your doctor will be your partner on your road to a healthy life. Don't settle for any less no matter what.

Keep Your Notebook/Journal Up to Date

Your notebook can become your biggest asset on your road to a healthy heart. We're all much too busy to remember every little detail about our lives—even when it's important. This notebook is your personal health bible. It contains everything—your family medical history, a list of your symptoms or complaints, medications, tests, allergies, and so on, and a record of what you asked and learned from your doctor. It's also a summary of the progress you've made in changing your diet, starting to exercise, and reducing your stress.

For example, if you were told you have high blood pressure, it would be helpful for you to have your blood pressure taken every few days while at the drugstore or supermarket. Record how you're feeling on that day along with your blood pressure reading. Don't forget to bring your log with you to your next doctor appointment.

If you were encouraged to lose weight and exercise, record your daily exercise activities in the log and your weight on a weekly basis. Also include how you are feeling when exercising and how your food intake has been. If you were encouraged to stop smoking, you can use your log to assist in this as well. Your log will become a valuable tool for you to share with your doctor and will assist in promoting good communication between both of you.

You don't need to write in it every day; once a week should be sufficient and whenever you encounter a major setback or success. Feel free to record anything else you don't want to forget, like the date of your next appointment, lab tests that need to be scheduled, and questions to ask the doctor either by phone or on your next visit.

Get into the Habit of Taking Care of Yourself

It's not uncommon to feel nervous, embarrassed, or even scared (or all of the above), especially if it's the first time you've gone to the doctor in years or if you are seeing a new doctor. Don't let these feelings overwhelm you. It's important that you remember why you scheduled the appointment. You want to stay healthy and you want to have problems diagnosed early so you know how to control or eliminate them and stay free of heart disease. Heart disease is a particular threat to women of color. So never put off seeing your doctor or having your regular testing done. Your life may depend on it.

In Case of an Emergency

If you do have health problems or you take medication, keep important medical information with you at all times. Keep a list of your current health problems (diabetes, high blood pressure, allergies, and so on) and the name and dosage of medications you take on a piece of paper in your wallet. Also include your doctor's name and phone number. Additionally you can register for a Medical Alert bracelet. The bracelet or the list can speed your treatment when it's needed. Several Web sites that offer medical alert bracelets: www.medicalert.org and www.americanmedical-id.com.

Signs of a Heart Attack

The "typical" female presentation of signs and symptoms of heart attack can be more complex and less classic than those of men. While men and women share many similar symptoms for heart attack, women tend to have a broader range of signs of heart disease that include less classic findings. Women are more likely than men to have "silent" or unrecognized heart attacks. Not all heart attacks begin with sudden, crushing chest pain, as we often see on TV or in the movies.

Women are more likely than men to have nausea, pain high up in the abdomen, or burning in their chest during a heart attack. Heart attack symptoms may be severe from the start, or they may be mild at first and then gradually worsen.

When to Call 911

If you feel any of the following symptoms that last for two minutes or more, call 911 or go to an emergency room—whichever will get you assistance faster:

- pressure, fullness, or squeezing pain in the center of your chest
- tightness, burning, or aching under your breastbone
- chest pain with light-headedness, shortness of breath, and sweating

Major symptoms *prior to* a heart attack may include:

- unusual fatigue
- sleep disturbance
- shortness of breath

- indigestion
- anxiety

Major symptoms *during* a heart attack include:

- shortness of breath
- weakness
- unusual fatigue
- cold sweats
- dizziness

As the medical community continues to study the differences between men and women who have heart attacks, it is becoming more clear that women's symptoms are not as predictable as men's.

Time is a crucial factor in a heart attack. Within the first few hours of arriving at the emergency room, drugs that break down blockage in the arteries (clot-busting drugs called thrombolytics) can be given to limit the size of the heart attack and prevent extensive damage to the heart muscle. Therefore, it is important not to miss the earliest possible opportunity to prevent or limit the size of a heart attack.

Always remember that heart disease and heart attacks can be prevented or controlled by making even small changes in the way you live. A healthy heart requires a personal action plan, starting with a complete medical checkup as a sensible first step. Beginning your heart-healthy plan, especially if you have multiple risk factors, is also crucial. Finally, partnering with your doctor is important in leading a heart-healthy life and controlling risk factors to prevent heart disease and heart attacks.

> *I think it is important for every woman to decide to be healthy, to be wise and to be kind.*
>
> —MAYA ANGELOU

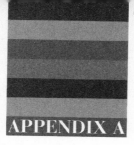

Resources for Heart-Smart Recipes

In combination with exercise and stress reduction, eating well is an excellent way to boost heart health. As discussed in Chapter 7, some of the changes you need to make are in what you eat and how much you eat.

Eating less fat (especially saturated fat), cholesterol, and salt (sodium) can make a difference. The following resources will assist you in finding a variety of heart-healthy recipes that can be purchased for a small cost or downloaded free off the Web sites. We know some are likely to become your family's favorites!

The Cost of Eating Heart Healthy

We realize that eating heart healthy on a limited budget can be as challenging as selecting the new and different foods. The cost of heart-healthy food items can be a consideration for many women who are preparing the meals and often balancing the checkbook too. Try to make as many heart-healthy choices as possible and incorporate them into your daily diet. The long-term investment that you are making for yourself and your family—health—is priceless.

What's Cooking?

Go to the following Web sites to find recipes for heart-healthy meals. You may print some sample recipes for free or even download an entire pamphlet or brochure. Add them to your loose-leaf binder divided into sections by meals—breakfast, lunch, dinner, snacks.

American Heart Association, www.americanheart.org

Look for the publications section. You will find a magazine cookbook link, which has several cookbooks that provide heart-healthy recipes. Choose from *Healthy Soul Food Recipes, Love Your Heart,* and *Healthy Recipes Kids Love,* which will help your children join in and have some fun. The publications will make preparing dishes at home easy, delicious, and heart healthy.

National Heart, Lung and Blood Institute, www.nhlbi
.nih.gov

One selection you may enjoy looking at is "Stay Young
at Heart," which has recipes such as Curtido Cabbage Sal-
vadore, Oven-Fried Yucca, Good-for-You Cornbread, and
Homestyle Biscuits. They offer *Delicious Heart Healthy
Latino Recipes* that can be purchased or downloaded and
printed at home or your local library. This bilingual cookbook has twenty-three tested recipes that cut down on saturated fat, cholesterol, and sodium but not on taste. These
delicious recipes are destined to become family favorites.

WomenHeart, www.womenheart.org

Click on the section called "Heart Healthy Recipes."
You will find more than twenty free recipes that you can
print out and try with your friends and family.

If you are doing our heart-smart program with a group of
girlfriends, you may want to share recipes. Before you
know it, you will have a loose-leaf binder filled with recipes
and comments from the group—a valuable resource.

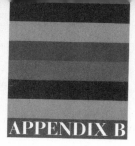

Helpful Health-Care Facts

Health care is expensive if you don't have health insurance, aren't old enough for Medicare, or make too much money for Medicaid coverage but not enough to pay for doctor visits, therapy, and medications. If you fall into any of these categories, discuss this with the doctor's office and work out a payment schedule or a fee adjustment based on your income. Most doctors are willing to do this, but if you don't ask, you'll never know. If you can't afford the cost of health-care coverage at all, there are ways to get the care you need.

Emergency Care

If you have no insurance and no money, anyone who comes to a hospital's emergency department asking for examination or treatment for a medical condition must be examined to determine if it's an emergency, according to the Federal Emergency Medical Treatment and Active Labor Act (EMTALA), also known as COBRA or the Patient Anti-Dumping Law. If it's an emergency, the hospital is required either to provide free treatment until you are stable or transfer you to another hospital. Almost every hospital in the country (except for some military hospitals and Shriner's hospitals) must comply with this rule.

It's important, however, that you don't use the emergency room as your "regular physician." An emergency room is to be used only in the case of an emergency, such as suffering a severe heart attack. Even if your family has no money or no insurance, never hesitate to go to the ER. They cannot turn you away and are required by law to examine and treat you, or transfer you for treatment to another hospital.

Medicaid

If your income is below a certain amount, you may already know about Medicaid, the state-run public health program that covers health care and transportation. States must cover some benefits, including hospital and outpatient care, doctor services, and home health services. More information about eligibility at your local welfare and medical assistance offices will tell you exactly what's covered where you live and what the income limits are, because this is different from state to state. More information about Medicaid is available at www.CMS.gov.

Medication Costs

By far the most expensive aspect of becoming ill is the cost of medication. If you don't have insurance or your plan doesn't include a prescription drug benefit, some drug companies provide free samples of medications to doctors, and many offer these samples free to their patients. If you can't afford any medication, ask your doctor whether any samples are available.

Other Insurance Resources

Check on your state's Web site; many states offer programs for the uninsured, especially for children.

You also may be surprised to know that some drug companies offer free medications directly to patients who can't afford them. You can apply for these patient assistance programs, usually with a doctor's note, along with proof of financial need or a statement that you or your family has no health insurance or prescription drug benefit. Speak to your doctor or nurse-practioner for more details.

Clinics

Call your local hospital and ask if they have a clinic. The range of services available in each clinic will vary. Contact the clinic you are interested in visiting first to find out the type of services they offer as well as the location and hours they are available.

Community Health Centers

Many community health centers provide health-care services to the uninsured on a sliding fee scale. This means that the fee charged to you for your care is based on your income.

Places of Worship

Many churches and other places of worship have resources available to assist uninsured members. You may want to call and ask if they can help you locate a doctor or clinic for health-care services. Places of worship often serve as a host for a mobile van that can provide health-care services to their congregation.

Patient Assistance Programs Web Sites

Individual drug companies often list their own programs online, so you can search for a company's name and check out its Web site. To make things easier, you can go to any of the Web sites listed below; they provide information about many different patient assistance programs providing free prescription medications to eligible participants. If you do not have access to a computer, all public libraries have computers for free public use.

Free Medicine Foundation
www.freemedicinefoundation.com/
Established by volunteers, Free Medicine Foundation has helped countless families across the nation completely eliminate or substantially reduce their prescription drug bills. Last year, these programs helped an estimated 7.6 million patients fill more than 11 million prescriptions. Free Medicine Foundation is designed to help patients nationwide obtain free prescription drugs. Those without prescription coverage, a low income, or maxed-out prescription benefits are encouraged to apply. Families with incomes ranging from below the national poverty level up to $38,000 (and in some cases, families with annual incomes as high as $60,000) can receive free drugs. Each sponsored drug has its own eligibility criteria.

The Medicine Program
www.themedicineprogram.com/
Through a special discount available only to large groups and corporations, this program offers a unique discount prescription drug program. Everyone is eligible. Membership is

absolutely free of charge and is available to anyone looking to lower the cost of his or her prescription bills. Visit the Web site to print a free prescription card, present it at over 35,000 participating pharmacies, and save up to 60 percent on medication.

NeedyMeds
120 Western Avenue
Gloucester, MA 01930
www.needymeds.com
NeedyMeds is a source of information on patient assistance programs and other programs that help people obtain health supplies and equipment. Information is always available at this site at no cost. It continues to grow with new information and links. In response to requests for printed versions of the data, the *NeedyMeds Manual* is now offered for sale, which contains the information on the Web site for those who find it easier to use a printed version rather than accessing the Web site.

Partnership for Prescription Assistance
1-888-4PPA-NOW (1-888-477-2669)
www.pparx.org/Intro.php
The partnership combines pharmaceutical companies, doctors, other health-care providers, patient advocacy organizations, and community groups to help qualifying patients who lack prescription coverage get the medicines they need through the public or private program that's right for them.

Many people qualify for free or nearly free medications. Among the organizations collaborating on this program are the American Academy of Family Physicians, the American Autoimmune Related Diseases Association, the Lupus Foundation of America, the NAACP, the National Alliance for Hispanic Health, and the National Medical Association.

RxAssist

www.rxassist.org

RxAssist offers a comprehensive database of patient assistance programs run by pharmaceutical companies to provide free medications to people who cannot afford to buy their medicine. The site also offers practical tools, news, and articles for health-care professionals and patients.

Help with Your Medications

As of late 2006, at least forty-one states had established or authorized some type of program to provide drug coverage or help primarily to low-income elderly or persons with disabilities who do not qualify for Medicaid, usually for people who meet certain enrollment criteria. Visit the National Conference of State Legislatures (NCSL) online at www.ncsl.org/programs/health/drugaid.htm.

7700 East First Place
Denver, CO 80230

Tel: 303-364-7700
Fax: 303-364-7800

444 North Capitol Street, NW, Suite 515
Washington, DC 20001
Tel: 202-624-5400
Fax: 202-737-1069

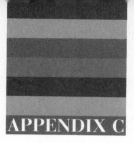

Common Heart Medications, Treatment, and Tests

Once heart disease has developed, there are several different ways to treat coronary artery disease, beginning with various types of medications. Some medicines decrease the workload on the heart, while others reduce the chance of having a heart attack or dying suddenly. Still others prevent or delay the need for a special procedure, such as angioplasty or by-pass surgery. Several types of medicine are commonly used.

Medications

ACE (angiotensin-converting enzyme) inhibitors help to lower blood pressure and reduce strain on your heart. They also may reduce the risk of a future heart attack and heart failure. Commonly used ACE inhibitors are: benazepril (Lotensin), captopril (Capoten), Enalapril (Vasotec), Lisinopril (Prinivil, Zestril), and ramipril (Altace).

Anticoagulants help to prevent clots from forming in your arteries and blocking blood flow. They include anisindione (Miradon), dicumarol, and warfarin (Coumadin).

Aspirin and other antiplatelets help to prevent clots from forming in your arteries and blocking blood flow. Aspirin may not be appropriate for some people, because it increases the risk of bleeding.

Beta-blockers slow your heart rate and lower your blood pressure to decrease the workload on your heart. They are used to relieve angina and may also reduce the risk of a future heart attack. Commonly used beta-blockers are atenolol (Tenormin), metoprolol (Lopressor), and propranolol (Inderal).

Calcium channel blockers relax blood vessels and lower blood pressure, ease the heart's workload, help widen coronary arteries, and relieve and control angina. Commonly used medications are amlodipine (Norvasc) and diltiazem (Cardizem).

Cholesterol-lowering medicines help to reduce your cholesterol to a doctor-recommended level. Commonly used cholesterol-lowering medications are the statins: simvastatin (Zocor), atorvastatin (Lipitor), rosuvastatin (Crestor), pravastatin (Pravachol). Others are Gemfibrozil (Lopid) and niacin/lovastatin (Advicor).

Long-acting nitrates are similar to nitroglycerin but are longer acting and can limit the occurrence of chest pain when used regularly over a long period. Commonly used nitrates are isosorbide dinitrate and nitroglycerin.

A recent clinical research study showed that African-American patients with heart failure who take a fixed-dose combination of the medications isosorbide dinitrate and hydralazine (BiDil) significantly decreased deaths from heart failure.

Nitroglycerin widens the coronary arteries, increasing blood flow to the heart muscle and relieving chest pain.

Invasive or Surgical Treatments

If medication doesn't take care of your particular problems, surgery or a cardiac intervention may be your only option. These treatments (angioplasty or bypass surgery) may be used to treat coronary artery disease if medications and lifestyle changes haven't improved your symptoms, or if your symptoms are getting worse.

Angioplasty and stent placement opens blocked or narrowed coronary arteries, improving blood flow to the heart, relieving chest pain, and possibly preventing a heart attack. Sometimes a device called a stent is placed in the artery to keep the artery open after the procedure.

Coronary artery bypass surgery. During this procedure, arteries or veins are taken from other places in your body to bypass narrowed coronary arteries. Bypass surgery can improve blood flow to the heart, relieve chest pain, and prevent a heart attack.

Your doctor may prescribe cardiac rehabilitation for angina or after bypass surgery, angioplasty, or a heart attack. Cardiac rehab can help you recover faster, feel better, and develop a healthier lifestyle. Almost everyone with coronary artery disease can benefit from cardiac rehab. Rehab usually includes exercise training and education.

Diagnosing Heart Disease

Although we presented a heart disease "risk quiz" at the beginning of this book, there really isn't a standard "heart disease test." If your doctor suspects heart disease, you'll be asked about your medical history and your family's health. Next, the doctor will check to see if you have any risk factors and do a physical exam. Based on the results of these preliminary procedures, your doctor may order an electrocardiogram (EKG), an echocardiogram, a stress test, or other diagnostic tests. These tests fall into two categories: noninvasive and invasive.

Noninvasive Tests

Blood tests. Your doctor may order a fasting glucose test to check your blood sugar level and a fasting lipoprotein profile to check your cholesterol levels.

Chest X-ray takes a picture of the organs and structures

inside the chest, including the heart, lungs, and blood vessels.
EKG (electrocardiogram) measures the rate and regularity of your heartbeat.

Heart-imaging tests. If your doctor needs more information than an exercise stress test can provide, stress testing is often combined with echocardiography (stress echo) or nuclear heart testing (stress nuclear scan).

Echocardiography uses sound waves to show blood flow through the chambers and valves of your heart and shows the strength of your heart muscle.

Nuclear heart scan uses a radioactive tracer and a special camera to evaluate the blood flow to the heart during exercise and at rest. A nuclear scan can indicate if there is scar tissue indicating that a heart attack occurred.

Stress test. Some heart problems are easier to diagnose when your heart is working harder and beating faster than when it's at rest. During exercise stress testing, your blood pressure and EKG readings are monitored while you walk or run on a treadmill or pedal a bicycle.

Invasive Test

Cardiac catheterization (coronary angiography) identifies possible problems with the arteries of the heart. A thin plastic tube is passed through an artery in the groin or arm to reach the coronary arteries. A special dye is injected into the tube so X-rays can show if you have any artery blockage or other heart problems.

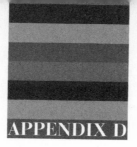

Questions and Answers About Heart Disease

Q. When can I resume sexual activity after a heart attack?
A. Although intimacy is an extremely important part of healing and living, you should look at it as any other physical activity you'll be resuming. Unless your doctor tells you otherwise, you may resume sexual activity as soon as you feel comfortable. Always start slowly, and if you become uncomfortable, stop—just like climbing stairs!

If you've had heart surgery and have an incision on your chest along the breastbone, you need to allow the bone and skin incision to heal. Sexual activity can be resumed slowly; you just need to be a bit more creative in terms of activities and positions and take it easy. It's also best to be the less active partner during sex and try to avoid placing pressure on your chest or breastbone.

Communication with your partner is crucial! Before resuming sexual activity, talk together about your feelings and fears. Your partner most likely has the same fears and concerns as you do.

Q. What about sexual positions after open-heart surgery?

A. A woman I spoke to long after her open-heart surgery said she was afraid to have intercourse again. Actually, I think the exact word she used was "terrified." "My breastbone was spread open like a chicken," she said. "How am I supposed to have intercourse again? I'm afraid that if I put pressure on my chest, it may cause the stitches to pop open."

The breastbone takes anywhere from six to ten weeks to heal. If you put significant pressure on the bone before it's healed, it may cause the bone to become unstable. If the bone isn't stable, it cannot "knit" together and will not heal properly. It's the same with the healing of any broken bone. Think about when you break a leg and you're in a cast for two months. The purpose of the cast is to keep the bone immobile.

We cannot put your chest in a cast, since it would make breathing very difficult. Instead, the bone is wired together with stainless steel sutures. These help keep the bone immobile until it heals completely. Once the breastbone is healed, your sexual position should not be of any concern.

Q. Is it safe to take an aspirin a day to prevent heart disease?

A. If you've already had a heart attack, low-dose aspirin (81 mg daily) helps to lower the risk of having another one, and recent studies also have shown that low-dose aspirin prevents stroke in women. Aspirin also helps to keep arteries open if you've had a heart bypass or other artery-opening procedure such as coronary angioplasty. But because of its risks, aspirin is *not* approved by the Food and Drug Administration for preventing heart attacks in healthy people. It may even be harmful for some people, especially those with no risk of heart disease. Talk to your doctor about whether taking aspirin is right for you. Be sure not to confuse aspirin with other common pain-relieving products such as acetaminophen (Tylenol), ibuprofen (Advil, Motrin), or naproxyn sodium (Aleve).

Aspirin is the only over-the-counter drug that has been shown to prevent heart attack or stroke. Although acetaminophen, ibuprofen, and naproxen sodium are, like aspirin, good drugs for pain and fever, only aspirin has demonstrated a beneficial effect for recurrent heart attack and stroke prevention.

Q. I heard that people with gum disease are at risk for heart disease. Is that true?

A. It's true. Researchers have found that people with gum disease are almost twice as likely to suffer from coronary artery disease as those without periodontal disease. There are several theories. First, many scientists believe that bacteria in the mouth can affect the heart by entering the bloodstream, attaching to fatty plaques in the heart blood vessels, and contributing to clot formation. Coronary artery disease is characterized by a thickening of the walls of the coronary arteries due to the buildup of cholesterol and other fatty compounds, calcium, and additional inflamatory substances. Blood clots can obstruct normal blood flow, restricting the amount of nutrients and oxygen required for the heart to function properly. This may lead to heart attacks. Another possibility is that the inflammation caused by periodontal disease increases plaque buildup, which may contribute to swelling of the arteries.

Periodontal disease also can worsen existing heart conditions. For example, patients at risk for infective endocarditis may require antibiotics before having any dental procedures. Your dentist and cardiologist will be able to determine if your heart condition requires use of antibiotics prior to dental procedures.

So practice good oral housekeeping: Brush twice a day and floss once every day. Have your teeth cleaned at least once a year (every six months is better).

Q. Do birth control pills and hormone replacement therapy (HRT) increase a woman's risk for heart disease?
A. The American Heart Association recommends that women should not be given HRT to prevent heart disease,

and that women with heart disease or who have had a stroke should not start taking hormones.

Menopause may increase a woman's risk for heart disease because it lowers levels of estrogen: For this reason, hormone replacement therapy (HRT) can work to ease symptoms of menopause by raising estrogen levels. This reduces common symptoms of menopause such as hot flashes and night sweats. It carries little increased risk of heart disease for pre-menopausal women (before menstrual periodsstop).

However, HRT *does* pose heart disease risks for women with high blood pressure and those who smoke. And while HRT can reduce the risk of heart disease for healthy women after menopause, it also increases the risk of other diseases, such as breast cancer.

Recent studies have shown that women who have gone through menopause and who have heart disease may have a higher risk of another cardiac problem—such as a heart attack—after starting HRT, at least in the short term. Women who have had a stroke have a higher risk of having another stroke if they start HRT.

Q. Is it okay to take vitamins and herbs for heart problems?
A. When it comes to vitamins and herbs, it's always best to check with both your pharmacist and your doctor before adding them to your daily regimen. There is a common mis-conception that because a prescription isn't needed for vita-

mins and herbs, they're always safe to take. That's certainly not the case! All drugs, whether over-the-counter or prescription, can interact with each other—some in a harmful way. This is why communication with your doctor and pharmacist is crucial. If you don't always use the same pharmacy for your prescription drugs, it's important to bring along a written list of every drug, herb, supplement, and vitamin you're taking. Drug interactions may not show up on the pharmacy computer if the list of what you're taking is incomplete.

So you can take vitamins and herbal remedies, **if your doctor and pharmacist know about them and they are certain there aren't any unpleasant side effects.** Be sure to take this list along whenever you go to a doctor, dentist, surgeon, nurse-practitioner, nutritionist, or hospital. Tell all of your health-care providers what you're taking. It's your responsibility to do so. Only then can they provide the proper health care.

Most doctors are not well informed about herbal remedies. This can be dangerous, because many herbs (even herbal teas) interact badly with some prescription medications. You can go to the People's Pharmacy Web site at www.peoplespharmacy.org/index.asp. Click on "Herb Library" in the left-hand column. Any herb you are taking is sure to be listed, and you can find out all about it.

Q. I had my heart fixed weeks ago. Why am I still so sad and tired?
A. Recent scientific studies have shown a strong link between depression and heart disease in women. Women who

are depressed are twice as likely to suffer heart problems, even in the absence of other risk factors. Also, women with coronary heart disease are twice as likely to die if they show symptoms of depression. Depression also makes it harder to control blood pressure.

A very high percentage of women (more than half) say they suffer depression, anxiety, or both as a result of heart disease—which may help explain why only a small fraction of women make lifestyle changes after their attack. If you're depressed, you're unlikely to have the incentive or energy to be able to make the necessary lifestyle changes to prevent another heart attack.

It needn't be that way. Depression is absolutely treatable and responds to a combination of medication and counseling more than 90 percent of the time. In addition, strong social support improves survival in depressed women with heart disease. You may not feel like it, but try to maintain social contacts.

Support and understanding from family and friends is crucial in the well-being of a woman with heart disease. Family and friends should be educated about all aspects about heart disease. Become an information magnet! Depression can be conquered, with a combination of social support, antidepressants, and therapy. Collect brochures from your doctor's office and get information from the American Heart Association or WomenHeart about living and coping with heart disease. Share this information with your family and friends so they know what to expect and how they can help in your recovery from a heart attack or surgery and how they can become a source of support.

Support groups are key. If you've done all that you feel you're capable of and you're still feeling depressed, seek out professional help. Don't hesitate to ask your doctor for a recommendation.

Q. What about going to a rehab or gym after a heart attack? My doctor never mentioned it. Is it too late now?
A. It's never to late to start exercise, and you don't need to join a gym to get the benefits of exercise on the heart. If you've had a heart attack or coronary heart surgery, cardiac rehabilitation is of great benefit. So ask your doctor and sign up! Studies have shown that after heart attacks and coronary heart surgery, women benefit from cardiac rehabilitation and have a better quality of life.

Aerobic exercise—exercise that increases your heart rate, such as walking, swimming, jogging, running—has been shown to decrease the incidence of heart disease and stroke. Brisk walking has been shown to decrease the incidence of heart attacks and death from heart disease in women. Therefore, a simple step or simple goal of incorporating walking into your daily life could prevent a heart attack.

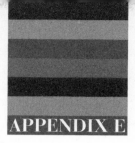

Women's Heart Centers

California

HeartMatters Program
Heart Care Center at Anaheim Memorial
1111 W. La Palma Avenue
Anaheim, CA 92801
714-999-6056
www.memorialcare.org/anaheim/services/heartmatters/
index.cfm

The physicians and staff at this center champion the prevention, diagnosis, and treatment of cardiovascular disorders in women. HeartMatters is a program for women that provides community education and outreach, free risk assessments, low-cost personal cardiac screenings, specialized in-hospital care, tobacco cessation program, and integrated vascular disease program. The program employs Spanish-speaking staff and physicians.

Women's Heart Institute
Cardiovascular Medical Group
414 N. Camden Drive, Suite 1100
Beverly Hills, CA 90210
310-278-3400
www.womensheartinstitute.com
This institute combines cardiovascular expertise with knowledge of women's health and gender-specific issues to produce a program that offers women maximum cardiovascular benefits.

Women's Cardiovascular Health Program and Clinic
Division of Cardiovascular Medicine
University of California Medical School
TB 172, One Shields Avenue
Davis, CA 95616
530-752-0717
www.ucdmc.ucdavis.edu/cardiology/wcvhp.html
A comprehensive program offering state-of-the-art cardiovascular health-care education services and studies on women's heart health issues. The program is staffed by a team of physicians and nurses at the UC Davis Medical Center and features the Women's Cardiovascular Medicine Clinic, providing dedicated care for women who are

at risk for or have heart disease. Physicians and nurse specialists use a multidisciplinary approach that emphasizes preventive measures and attention to heart issues unique to women. Because heart disease can be related to a variety of hereditary, lifestyle, and environmental factors, the clinic offers a wide range of preventive, diagnostic, risk assessment, treatment, educational, and referral services, including specialty cardiovascular medicine; primary care in women's health; risk factor analysis and intervention, including diagnosis and treatment of lipid disorders; gynecological evaluation and screening, including mammography and Pap smears; dietary intervention; smoking cessation; exercise training; stress reduction; patient educational sessions; women's mental health services; and participation in women's cardiovascular research studies at UC Davis.

San Fernando Valley Women's Heart Center
Tarzana-Encino Medical Center
16661 Ventura Boulevard, Suite 820
Encino, CA 91436
818-905-6110
This free-standing women's heart clinic offers a range of diagnostic testing, mental health assessment, and a variety of related services including nutrition counseling, weight management counseling, classes in smoking cessation and physical activity, cardiac rehab services, and community and patient education.

Women's Heart Center
St. Joseph Hospital of Orange
1140 W. La Veta Avenue
Orange, CA 92868
714-744-8791
www.sjo.org

This facility is dedicated solely to the prevention, early detection, and treatment of heart disease in women. It provides low-cost personal heart and vascular screenings; free heart and self-health risk assessments; educational seminars addressing nutrition, exercise, and osteoporosis; and specialized in-hospital care for women admitted with heart disease.

Florida

Women's Heart Care
Southwest Florida Heart Group
8540 College Parkway
Fort Myers, FL 33919
239-433-8879

The program's overall goal is to educate women, help change lifestyle habits, and prevent heart disease. The center offers a number of screenings, including blood pressure; body mass index; cholesterol; glucose; and abdominal, carotid artery, and echo imaging. The center considers an individual's specific risk to develop a personalized plan of action to minimize risk of heart attack or stroke.

Women's Heart Program
Cardiovascular Center of South Florida
7400 SW 87th Avenue, Suite 100
Miami, FL 33173
305-275-8200
www.heartworld.com/images/uploaded/heartworld/
women.cfm

This program is dedicated to the prevention, early detection, and treatment of heart disease in women and also provides education and support services. Each patient is evaluated by a cardiologist who has specialized training in women's heart care. In addition, the program offers Woman to Woman Networking for those who have experienced heart disease firsthand, which includes a support group and personalized "Heart Friend" who is there to help with recovery after a cardiac event. These very special women volunteers help patients make lifestyle changes while recovering from cardiovascular disease and are strong advocates that women experience heart disease differently from men.

Georgia

Women's Heart Center
Cardiovascular Centers of Georgia
755 Mt. Vernon Highway, Suite 530
Atlanta, GA 30328
404-832-7802
www.womensheartcenter.com

Part of the cardiology group project, the center offers a variety of diagnostic testing, treatments, mental health assessment, nutrition counseling, weight management counseling, support groups, smoking cessation classes, patient education, clinical research trials, physical activity counseling, and educational materials.

Illinois

The Bluhm Cardiovascular Institute of Northwestern Memorial Hospital's Center for Women's Cardiovascular Health
Feinberg Pavilion
251 E. Huron
Chicago, Illinois 60611
Toll-free: 866-662-8467

Founded on the principles of identifying cardiovascular disease in women of all ages and providing care that is designed specifically for women, the cardiovascular center is committed to meeting the needs of women affected by cardiovascular disease through a multidisciplinary team approach. The physicians at the center are dedicated to promoting women's awareness of cardiovascular health, addressing risk factors including stress, tobacco use, nutrition, and exercise, and are committed to conducting clinical trials to advance the knowledge of cardiovascular care for women.

The Center for Women's Cardiovascular Health is developing a standard of care that recognizes women as unique individuals and tailors treatment strategies to optimize their specific cardiovascular needs.

Women's Heart Center
Fox Valley Cardiovascular Consultants
2088 Ogden Avenue, Suite 180
Aurora, IL 60504
630-851-6440
www.womensheart.com

Established to help slow the escalating incidence of heart disease in women, the center offers innovative care in a unique, nurturing environment with specialists focused solely on women's heart care, providing a full range of preventive, diagnostic, and treatment options. Through support groups, educational programs, and screenings, the center offers preventative strategies to apply to women's daily routines. In addition, the center has partnered with an exercise center to offer cardiovascular fitness on-site. The Women's Heart Center is one of five centers in the country to receive a grant from the Office of Women's Health for the Advancement of Women's Awareness of cardiovascular Risk Education (AWARE) in the specialty setting program. The goal of the AWARE program is to reduce heart disease mortality and morbidity among women and increase the number of high-risk women receiving quality heart care.

Kansas

Women's Cardiovascular Center
Kramer & Crouse Cardiology, P.C.
7301 East Frontage Road, Suite 200
Shawnee Mission, KS 66204
913-432-7474

The center offers diagnostic testing and a range of services including patient education events, professional education, and clinical research trials.

Kentucky

Norton Suburban Women's Heart Center
Norton Healthcare
Medical Plaza III
4121 Dutchman's Lane, Suite 102
Louisville, KY 40207
502-899-6960
www.nortonhealthcare.com

The first center in the region devoted to heart disease awareness and prevention for women, offering a variety of programs and treatment options from comprehensive diagnostic procedures to innovative surgeries. The center offers research, screenings, education, awareness, and prevention programs to teach women how to lower their risks. The center offers a $40 heart disease risk screening, including a total lipid profile, cholesterol/HDL ratio, glucose, blood pressure, body fat analysis, and ankle-brachial index, as well as education on heart disease risk factors, lifestyle, and signs and symptoms of heart disease.

Louisiana

Women's Heart Program
Christus St. Frances Cabrini Hospital
3330 Masonic Drive
Alexandria, LA 71301
318-561-4172

Women's Heart Program
Our Lady of Lourdes Regional Medical Center
601 W. St. Mary's Boulevard, Suite 410
Lafayette, LA 70506
337-289-4673

Massachusetts

Center for Cardiovascular Disease in Women
Brigham and Women's Hospital
75 Francis Street
Boston, MA 02115
617-732-8985
www.brighamandwomens.org/ConnorsCenter/
cardiovascular/

The Center for Cardiovascular Disease in Women is dedicated to developing new sex- and gender-specific strategies for the prevention, treatment, and rehabilitation of coronary heart disease in women. The center is committed to improving and maintaining women's heart health through excellence in clinical care, research, patient and provider education, and community outreach and advocacy. Programs include *Sister Talk 2*, a ten-part cable television series designed to help viewers learn simple and practical strategies to improve their heart health, and *To the Heart of Women,* a cardiovascular disease prevention and risk reduction program for black and Latina women.

Michigan

Ministrelli Women's Heart Center
William Beaumont Hospital
3601 W. Thirteen Mile Road
Royal Oak, MI 48073
248-551-8794
www.beaumonthospitals.com/pls/portal30/site.web
_pkg.page?xpageid=mwhc_home

The Ministrelli Women's Heart Center is dedicated to the detection, prevention, and treatment of heart disease in women. This state-of-the-art facility offers on-site diagnostic capabilities including stress tests, EKGs, and echocardiograms (heart ultrasounds). The staff is dedicated to helping women get healthy and stay healthy.

McLaren's Heart and Vascular Women's Program
McLaren Regional Medical Center
G-3286 Beecher Road
Flint, MI 48532
810-720-3370

This free-standing women's heart clinic offers some diagnostic testing, referrals, management of cholesterol and obesity, nutrition and weight management counseling, classes on smoking cessation and exercise, support groups, patient education events, professional education, community education events, clinical research trials, wellness programs, and educational materials.

Minnesota

Mayo Clinic Women's Heart Clinic
Mayo Clinic Rochester
200 First Street SW
Rochester, MN 55981
507-284-3546
www.mayoclinic.org/cardiovascular-rst/womensclinic
.html

The Mayo Clinic has developed this heart clinic to treat and prevent heart disease while addressing the distinct concerns of women. Patients have full access to Mayo Clinic's state-of-the-art diagnostic, therapeutic, and surgical services, both for heart disease and other conditions that may be discovered. There are several components included in a visit to the Women's Heart Clinic, including risk assessment, comprehensive cardiac diagnostic evaluation, risk management, education, hormone therapy discussion, and coordinated care. A health-care professional guides each patient in making healthy lifestyle changes to help prevent or slow the progression of heart disease. Depending on the patient's unique needs, recommendations may include blood pressure measurement and control, personalized exercise prescription, healthy eating plan, smoking cessation advice, and stress management techniques. Women's Heart Clinic staff members understand women's unique heart risks and help patients and their home physicians manage their risks.

Missouri

Muriel I. Kauffman Women's Heart Center
Saint Luke's Mid America Heart Institute
4401 Wornall Road
Kansas City, MO 64111
816-932-5624
www.saintlukeshealthsystem.org/slhs/com/mahi/html/
patients/WomensCardiac/treatment/index.htm
The institute helps women understand their individual risks for heart disease by offering the latest information and services on the unique characteristics of women's cardiovascular health risk analysis from early diagnosis and treatment. A one-on-one interactive assessment screening focuses on overall cardiovascular health promotion and disease prevention,

while stimulating and empowering women to take a proactive role in their cardiovascular health. The Women's Heart Center is devoted to the hearts of women and cherishes the relationships, partnering, and opportunities to educate women about their vulnerability to heart disease and understand their individual risks by offering the latest information on cardiovascular health from risk analysis to early diagnosis and treatment. Its services are designed to complement the health care women receive from their personal physician.

Nebraska

Women's Heart Center
Alegent Health
16940 Lakeside Hills Plaza
Omaha, NE 68130
402-758-5265
www.nebraskamed.com/services/womens/index.aspx

New York

Total Heart Care, PC
177 East 87th Street, Suite 503
New York, NY 10128
212-289-2045
www.TotalHeartCare.com; www.NiecaGoldberg.com
Prevention, diagnosis, and treatment of heart disease and

related disorders, including risk-factor testing and management, diagnostic stress testing, and medication and behav-
ioral/lifestyle assessment and counseling. Nieca Goldberg,
M.D., of Total Heart Care is also the director of the Women's
Cardiovascular Center at New York University.

Women's Healthy Heart Initiative
Albany Medical Center
47 New Scotland Avenue, MC 44
Albany, NY 12208
518-262-6766
Part of a multispecialty clinic, the center offers EKG, peripheral vascular ankle-bracelet index screening, and echocardiogram, along with some mental health assessments and
management of diabetes, high cholesterol, high blood pressure, obesity, and osteoporosis.

Women's Institute for Cardiovascular Care
Long Island Institute for Cardiovascular Care
206 Fallwood Parkway
Farmingdale, NY 11743
516-249-1020

Women's Institute for Cardiovascular Care
Huntington Heart Center
96 East Main Street
Huntington, NY 11743
631-385-0022

The institute offers a variety of diagnostic testing; mental health assessments; management of high cholesterol, hypertension, and obesity; as well as nutrition counseling, weight management counseling, and exercise counseling.

Women's Heart Program at the Strong Heart and Vascular Center
University of Rochester Medical Center—Strong Memorial Hospital
2400 S. Clinton Avenue
Building G, 1st Floor
Rochester, NY 14618
585-341-7791
www.stronghealth.com/services/cardiology/women/overview.cfm

Dedicated to promoting women's heart health and helping women lead healthy lives, this team of women physicians and health-care providers understands the special needs, concerns, and questions about heart disease facing women today. The program offers comprehensive cardiovascular evaluation, emphasizing early detection and prevention strategies to improve women's lifelong health and well-being. The center partners with obstetricians, gynecologists, and primary care providers to offer patients comprehensive diagnostic testing and treatment, which also encompasses treating women during life stages such as childbirth and menopause. As part of the Strong Heart and Vascular Center, the Women's Heart Program has access to the most comprehensive cardiovascular care in upstate New York. Women who participate in major drug and device trials have access to the newest medications and cardiac care before they become widely available.

North Carolina

UNC Women's Heart Program
UNC Health Care Chapel Hill North Medical Center
1838 Airport Avenue, Suite B19
Chapel Hill, NC 27514
919-929-4929

The Women's Heart Program seeks to educate, identify, and treat (if necessary) women of all ages at risk for cardiovascular disease. The center provides a pleasant atmosphere where education, diagnosis, and management can be efficiently addressed. The clinic offers expert physician care, lipid counseling, and diagnostic testing on-site. Two blocks away, the UNC Wellness Center offers dietary and exercise expertise including a certified cardiac rehabilitation program.

Pennsylvania

Woman, Infant and Fetal Heart Program
Magee-Womens Hospital
University of Pittsburgh Medical Center
300 Halket Street
Pittsburgh, PA 15213

412-647-4747

http://magee.upmc.com/HeartProgram.htm

Committed to enhancing women's health care through excellence in clinical care and leadership in the community, Magee, in partnership with the UPMC Cardiovascular Institute, has developed a comprehensive program to serve women, infants, and the fetus with or at risk for developing cardiovascular disease.

York Hospital Women's Heart Program
York Hospital Wellspan Health System
25 Monument Road, Suite 199
York, PA 17403
717-851-6000
www.wellspan.org/HealthServices/wellspanhfw
_womensheartprogram.htm

A hospital-based program that provides prevention, diagnosis, and treatment services for women who are at increased risk for cardiovascular disease or are known to have or suspected of having the disease. Each woman is evaluated for risk factors by a cardiologist who specializes in women's heart care, along with a nurse educator. An individualized plan of care can be designed to prevent a first heart attack or progression of existing heart disease. The program offers a free heart risk assessment to determine overall heart health and uses these results, if necessary, to make arrangements for a consultation and a heart disease prevention plan. The program also offers nutrition and weight management counseling, smoking cessation classes, support groups, cardiac rehab services, patient education events, professional education, community education events, physical activity counseling, wellness programs, and clinical research trials.

Rhode Island

Women's Cardiac Center at the Miriam Hospital Lifespan
164 Summit Avenue
Providence, RI 02906
401-793-7870
www.lifespan.org/tmh/services/cardiac/programs/
women/

Offers complete diagnostic and clinical cardiology services, cardiovascular surgery, and cardiac rehabilitation to women. Each new patient has a baseline evaluation, which includes a review of medical history, a cardiovascular physical examination, and an EKG, followed by an evaluation by a behavioral medicine specialist who can help the patient modify her lifestyle if necessary. Based on the patient's evaluation and interview, an individualized regimen of medications, diet, exercise, nutritional counseling, and stress management is provided. If necessary, a referral for noninvasive or invasive testing will be made. The center forwards the results and recommendations for each patient to her primary care physician.

Tennessee

Vanderbilt Women's Heart Center

Vanderbilt University Medical Center

2311 Pierce Avenue

Nashville, TN 37232

615-322-2318

This hospital-based program offers a variety of diagnostic testing, mental health assessments, management of high cholesterol and high blood pressure, as well as nutrition counseling, weight management counseling, clinical research trials, and exercise counseling.

Texas

Her Healthy Heart

St. Luke's Episcopal Hospital and Texas Heart Institute

6720 Bertner

Houston, TX 77030

832-355-5500

www.herhealthyheart.com

Her Healthy Heart is the only comprehensive women's heart program in Houston. Every patient is seen by an experienced nurse-practitioner acquainted with the full range of diagnostic and treatment options. The center offers body composition analysis, blood pressure evaluation, laboratory work, and other noninvasive tests.

Helpful Heart Organizations

The following organizations offer information about heart disease, heart health, heart-healthy living, and support.

American Diabetes Association
National Call Center
1701 North Beauregard Street
Alexandria, VA 22311
1-800-DIABETES or 1-800-342-2383
www.diabetes.org/
The nation's leading nonprofit health organization, providing diabetes research, information, and advocacy.

American Heart Association
National Center
7272 Greenville Avenue
Dallas, TX 75231
888-MY HEART
www.americanheart.org/simplesolutions
The mission of the AHA is to reduce disability and death from cardiovascular diseases and stroke. The organization offers useful information for African-American and Latina women about heart disease. Two useful and user-friendly programs to get you started in living a heart healthy lifestyle are Go Red for Women, information for women about heart disease, and Choose to Move, a twelve-week program for women to get started living a heart-healthy lifestyle.

The Association of Black Cardiologists
www.abcardio.org/women.htm
The Association of Black Cardiologists, Inc., (ABC) is dedicated to eliminating the disparities related to cardiovascular disease in all people of color.

Healthfinder
www.healthfinder.gov
Sponsored by the U.S. Department of Health and Human Services, this site offers Internet links to hundreds of sites that provide reliable consumer health-care information and support.

Institute for Healthcare Improvement
www.ihi.org/IHI/Topics/PatientCenteredCare/
ResourcesforPatientsandFamilies
Resources for patients who are looking for support after a particular medical event or who are trying to communicate with other patients and families about similar issues.

MEDLINEplus
http://medlineplus.gov
MEDLINEplus has extensive information from the National Institutes of Health and other trusted sources on more than 650 diseases and conditions, medications, and wellness issues.

National Council for Patient Information and Education
4915 Saint Elmo Avenue, Suite 505

Bethesda, MD 20814-6082

301-656-8565

www.talkaboutrx.com

A coalition of more than 125 diverse organizations whose mission is to stimulate and improve communication of information on appropriate medicine use to consumers and health-care professionals. NCPIE is the nation's leading authority for informing the general public and health-care professionals on safe medicine use through better communication.

National Heart, Lung and Blood Institute
Health Information Center
PO Box 30105

Bethesda, MD 20824-0105

301-592-8573

TTY: 240-629-3255

www.hearttruth.gov

NHLBI provides leadership for a national program in diseases of the heart, blood vessels, lungs, and blood; blood resources; and sleep disorders. NHLBI also has administrative responsibility for the NIH Woman's Health Initiative.

National Latina Health Network
www.nlhn.net

The National Latina Health Network is a growing network of individuals and organizations dedicated to improving the quality of health among Latinas and their families.

National Patient Safety Foundation

www.npsf.org/html/psaw.html

Tools and resources to help patients become active members of their health-care team. Educational activities are centered on educating patients on how to become involved in their own health care, as well as working with hospitals to build partnerships with their patient community.

National Women's Health Information Center

8270 Willow Oaks Corporate Drive

Fairfax, VA 22031

(800) 994-9662

www.womenshealth.gov

The federal government's source for information on women's health. Here you can access thousands of publications and organizations with information on hundreds of health topics. Trained English- and Spanish-speaking information and referral specialists will order free health information or provide organizational referrals to assist you with any health questions. NWHIC's phone lines are open Monday through Friday, 9 A.M. to 6 P.M. EST (excluding federal holidays).

Office on Women's Health

U.S. Department of Health and Human Services

National Women's Health Information Center

200 Independence Avenue SW, Room 712E

Washington, DC 20201

202-690-7650

Toll-free: 800-994-WOMAN

TDD: 1-888-220-5446

www.4woman.gov

This office partners with organizations to develop programs to stem the risk of cardiovascular disease in women. OWH works to improve the health and well-being of women and girls in the United States through its innovative programs, by educating health professionals, and by motivating behavior change in consumers through the dissemination of health information.

WomenHeart—The National Coalition for Women with Heart Disease

818 18th Street NW, Suite 930

Washington, DC 20006

tel: 202-728-7199

fax: 202-728-7238

www.womenheart.org

WomenHeart is the only national patient advocacy organization, serving the eight million women living with heart disease. It provides support, information, and advocacy to improve their quality of life and health care, including early detection, accurate diagnosis, and proper treatment. The group offers community-based support networks in nearly forty communities across America that provide a variety of services to women heart survivors, as well as national educational seminars and membership conferences. Free monthly email newsletter provides up-to-date information on program activities, as well as gender-specific cardiac medical research and information. Fitness and wellness resources provide helpful information on quitting smoking, exercising, and eating for a healthy heart. The online store provides books and other items for sale.

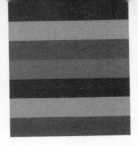

Glossary

aneurysm. A weak area on an artery that has ballooned out from the wall and filled with blood.

angina. Chest pain caused by a shortage of blood and oxygen to the heart.

angioplasty. A procedure in which a device with a small balloon on the tip of a catheter is inserted into a blood vessel to open up a blocked area. Lasers may be used to help break up the plaque. Catheters also may have spinning wires or drill tips to clean out the plaque.

anticoagulants. Drugs used to prevent the formation of blood clots.

antigen. A substance recognized as foreign by the immune system.

aorta. The main artery of the heart that begins at the opening of the heart's lower left chamber.

arrhythmia. An abnormal heart rhythm.

arteriogram. An X-ray of the arteries and veins that uses a special dye that can detect blockage or narrowing of the vessels. Also called an angiogram.

arteriosclerosis. A general term for the hardening and thickening of the arterial walls.

artery. Blood vessel that carries blood from the heart to other parts of the body.

atherosclerosis. A type of arteriosclerosis in which the artery walls thicken and narrow due to the buildup of cholesterol, restricting blood flow and leading to a heart attack or a stroke.

atria. The heart's two upper chambers. The right atrium receives blood directly from a vein. The left atrium receives oxygenated blood from the lungs.

atrial fibrillation. Irregular beating of the left upper chamber of the heart when electrical signals are fired in a very fast and uncontrolled manner.

body mass index (BMI). A measure of body fat based on height and weight that applies to both adult men and women. BMI categories: underweight=<18.5; normal weight=18.5–24.9; overweight=25–29.9; obesity=30 or greater.

capillary. Thin-walled tube that carries blood between arteries and veins.

cardiac arrest. A condition in which the heart stops beating.

cardiac perfusion imaging. A noninvasive diagnostic procedure in which dye is injected into the bloodstream and collects in the wall of the heart, used to assess the heart's blood flow or heart attack damage.

cardiomyopathy. A disease of the heart muscle in which the heart loses its ability to pump blood, leading to disturbed heart rhythm and irregular heartbeats.

cardiovascular disease (CVD). Any abnormal condition of the heart or blood vessels, including coronary heart disease, stroke, congestive heart failure, peripheral vascular disease, congenital heart disease, endocarditis, and many other conditions.

carotid artery. The artery located on either side of the neck that supplies the brain with blood.

carotid endarterectomy. Surgery used to remove fatty deposits from the carotid arteries.

catheterization, cardiac. An examination of the heart by threading a thin tube into a vein or artery and passing it into the heart to sample oxygen levels, measure pressure, or take an X-ray.

cholesterol. A waxy substance produced naturally by the liver that circulates in the blood and helps maintain tissues and cell membranes. Cholesterol is found throughout the body, including the nervous system, muscle, skin, liver, intestines, and heart. Too much cholesterol can contribute to atherosclerosis and high blood pressure.

congestive heart failure. The inability of the heart to deliver an adequate blood flow, because of heart disease or high blood pressure. When this occurs, blood backs up into the veins leading to the heart, causing breathlessness, salt and water retention, and swelling.

coronary arteries. Two arteries that travel from the aorta over the top of the heart, providing blood to the heart.

coronary artery disease (CAD). A condition caused by narrowed coronary arteries (atherosclerosis) that decreases the supply of blood to the heart (myocardial ischemia). Also known as ischemic heart disease.

diaphragm. The dome-shaped muscle located at the bottom of the lungs, used in breathing.

diastolic blood pressure. The lower number in a blood pressure reading that represents the pressure inside the arteries when the heart is filling up with blood between contractions.

diuretic. A medication that increases the rate that urine is produced, promoting the excretion of salts and water.

echocardiography. A diagnostic technique using ultrasound waves to image the interior of the heart.

electrocardiogram. A cardiovascular test that records the electrical impulses produced by the heart.

enzyme. A protein that causes or speeds up chemical reactions in the body; enzymes build up or synthesize most compounds in the body.

heart attack. A condition that occurs when a section of the heart doesn't get enough oxygenated blood and dies, caused by blockage of one or more of the coronary arteries.

heart failure. Death of heart muscle, causing loss of blood circulation and possibly death.

high-density lipoproteins (HDL). So-called good cholesterol containing mostly protein and less cholesterol and triglycerides; high levels are associated with lower risk of coronary heart disease.

homocysteine. An amino acid that occurs normally in the body. In high levels, homocysteine may increase a person's chances of developing heart disease and stroke.

hypertension. High blood pressure.

infarct. An area of tissue that is dead or dying because of a loss of blood supply.

ischemia. Decline in blood supply.

lipids. Fatty substances (including cholesterol and triglycerides) that are found in blood and tissues.

low-density lipoproteins (LDL). So-called bad cholesterol; high levels are associated with increased risk of coronary heart disease.

myocardial infarction. Heart attack.

myocardial ischemia. Lack of oxygen-carrying blood in an area of heart tissue due to blocked coronary arteries. Myocardial ischemia can cause chest pain, but it also can be painless. Without intervention, myocardial ischemia can lead to a heart attack.

nuclear stress test. Uses a radioactive tracer and a special camera to evaluate the blood flow to the heart during exercise and at rest. A nuclear scan can indicate if there is scar tissue indicating that a heart attack occurred.

oxygen-free radicals. Toxic chemicals released during the process of cellular respiration and released in excessive amounts as a cell dies.

pacemaker. An electrical device that controls the heartbeat and heart rhythm by emitting a series of electrical charges.

plaque. The buildup of fatty substances, cholesterol, cellular waste products, calcium, and fibrin (a clotting material in the blood) in the lining of an artery.

platelet. A colorless disk-shaped body in blood that aids clotting.

protein. Amino acid compound that the body uses for growth and repair. Foods that supply the body with protein include animal products, grains, legumes, and vegetables.

pulmonary artery. Artery carrying deoxygenated blood from the heart to the lungs.

saturated fat. Fat found in dairy products and meat; contributes to raised cholesterol levels.

stent. A tiny, expandable coil that is placed inside a blood vessel at the site of a blockage and then expanded to open up the blockage.

stroke. Loss of muscle function, vision, sensation, or speech caused by either a hemorrhage or an insufficient supply of blood to part of the brain, often due to narrowing of the arteries supplying blood to the brain. The hemorrhage may involve bleeding into the brain itself or the space around the brain.

systolic blood pressure. The top number in a blood pressure reading that is a measure of the pressure inside the arteries as the heart contracts.

total serum cholesterol. A combined measurement of a person's high-density lipoprotein (HDL) and low-density lipoprotein (LDL).

triglycerides. Fats carried through the bloodstream to tissues. Most of the body's fat is stored in the form of triglycerides for later use. Triglycerides are obtained primarily from fat in foods.

unsaturated fat. Fat that is usually liquid at room temperature; protects against heart disease.

valve. An opening between two chambers of the heart, or between a heart chamber and a blood vessel. When a heart valve is closed, no blood should leak through.

ventricles. The two lower heart chambers.

ventricular fibrillation. Electrical signals in the ventricles that are fired in a very fast and uncontrolled manner, causing the heart to quiver rather than beat and pump blood.

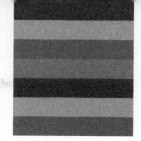

Suggested Reading

Books

The African-American Women's Guide to a Healthy Heart, Anne L. Taylor, MD, Hilton Publishing Company and the Association of Black Cardiologists Center for Women's Health (2004)

Cholesterol Down: Ten Simple Steps to Lower Your Cholesterol in Four Weeks—Without Prescription Drugs, Janet Bond Brill, PhD, Three Rivers Press (2006)

From the Heart: A Woman's Guide to Living Well with Heart Disease, Kathy Kastan, LCSW, MAEd, Da Capo Press (2007)

The Healthy Heart Handbook for Women, Marian Sandmaier, National Institutes of Health and National Heart, Lung and Blood Institute (2006)

Mayo Clinic Heart Book Second Edition, Mayo Foundation for Medical Education and Research (2000)

No-Fad Diet, American Heart Association, Clarkson/Potter Publishers (2005)

Stories from the Heart: Women Heart Patients Describe Their Disease, Treatment and Recovery, compiled and arranged by Anastasia Roussos and Melissa Lausin. WomenHeart: The National Coalition for Women with Heart Disease (2003)

Thriving with Heart Disease, Wayne M. Sotile, PhD, with Robin Cantor Cooke, Free Press (2003)

Women Are Not Small Men, Nieca Goldberg, MD, Ballantine Publishing Group (2002)

Magazines

Cooking Light
Web address: www.cookinglight.com

Heart-Healthy Living
Web address: www.hearthealthyonline.com

Prevention
Web address: www.prevention.com

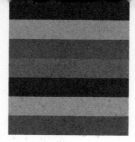

Index

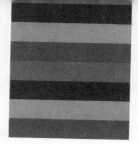

About the Authors

Jennifer H. Mieres, M.D., F.A.C.C., F.A.H.A.

Jennifer H. Mieres, M.D., F.A.C.C., F.A.H.A., a native of Trinidad, West Indies, is an associate professor of medicine and the director of Nuclear Cardiology at the Leon H. Charney Division of Cardiology at New York University School of Medicine. She is a nationally recognized expert in cardiovascular diseases in women and is routinely called upon by the media to comment on heart health. She has appeared on national and local media outlets including two recent documentaries for PBS entitled *A Woman's Heart* (2001) and *Call to Action: Women and Heart Disease* (2004).

A graduate of Bennington College and Boston University

School of Medicine, she is a Fellow of the American College of Physicians, American College of Cardiology (ACC), the American Society of Nuclear Cardiology (ASNC), and the American Heart Association (AHA), and is board certified in cardiovascular diseases and nuclear cardiology. Her society memberships also include the Association of Black Cardiologists and the American Medical Women's Association. She is a founding member and president-elect of the ASNC. She has presented her research papers on cardiovascular disease in women at national and international conferences and has been one of the distinguished faculty at scientific sessions of the AHA, ACC, and ASNC.

Dr. Mieres is a national spokesperson for the AHA and has served on the national board of directors (2004–2006) and was president of the board of directors (2003–2005) of the AHA's Long Island region. She is actively involved in community service and has been a guest speaker at several local and national community functions. She serves on the advisory board for WomenHeart (the national coalition for women living with heart disease).

In 2002, Dr. Mieres received the New York State Governor's Award for Excellence, and as a producer of *A Woman's Heart,* she was nominated for an Emmy for Best Documentary in the Health Science category at the 46th Annual New York Emmy Awards held in March 2003. In August of 2003, Dr. Mieres was featured as an "Everyday Hero" in *Newsday.* In 2004, she was awarded the WomenHeart Wenger Award for Healthcare, and in 2005, Dr.

Mieres received the Long Island American Heart Association Award for Outstanding Service as President of the Long Island Region and was the recipient of the Long Island American Heart Association William Groom Award for Volunteer of the Year.

Dr. Mieres is married to Dr. Haskel Fleishaker and lives in New York City with their daughter, Zöe.

Terri Ann Parnell, R.N., M.A.

Terri Ann Parnell was born in Brooklyn, New York, and grew up in Wantagh, Long Island. She began her professional career at St. Vincent's Hospital in New York City as a critical care nurse and moved to North Shore University Hospital in Manhasset, Long Island. She is currently the director of Cardiac Services for the North Shore–Long Island Jewish Health System.

Ms. Parnell is a nursing graduate of St. Vincent's Hospital School of Nursing in New York City. Her BSN was completed at Adelphi University in Garden City, New York. She went on to complete her master's degree in health care administration at Hofstra University in Hempstead, New York, where she served as an adjunct professor. Terri is currently pursuing her doctoral degree in nursing at Case Western Reserve University in Cleveland, Ohio.

Ms. Parnell lectures on patient education and women and heart disease. She is a member of Sigma Theta Tau, the Health Care Education Association, and is actively involved with the American Heart Association by whom she has been honored for her efforts in conjunction with the Long Island Heart Walk and the Go Red for Women Initiative. She has received nursing awards for excellence in research and patient and family education.

Ms. Parnell currently resides in Garden City, New York, with her husband and their children.

Carol A. Turkington

Carol A. Turkington is a medical writer and the author of more than fifty nonfiction books. A veteran journalist specializing in women's health, she has worked as a medical writer and an editor at Duke University Medical Center, and as senior writer in biobehavioral medicine at the American Psychological Association in Washington, D.C.

A freelance writer and editorial consultant for the past sixteen years, her clients have included the national office of the American Red Cross, Nestlé Foods, Hallmark, Nickelodeon, and a wide range of physicians and psychologists.